The EVERYTHING® Reiki Book

Dear Reader:

Whether you have already taken a Reiki class or you are just beginning to explore this natural hands-on healing system, it is my hope that this book will provide you with a broad-ranging scope and a clear understanding of the many nuances that collectively give Reiki its gentle healing power.

I am delighted to be able to play a contributing role in your exploration of Reiki through *The Everything® Reiki Book*. My personal journey with Reiki began in January 1996 when I participated in a Reiki Shiki Ryoho class under the careful direction of Usui Reiki Master/Teacher Reverend Beverley Jean Voss. Before that time, I was already walking the path of a holistic healer. I am always seeking to gain more healing knowledge and am often looking to add more tools to my healer's medicine bag. Reiki turned out to be an ideal complementary tool. Its constant availability, easy access, and great adaptability assist me regularly in treating others, as well as in my never-ending quest for personal well-being and spiritual growth. I am very pleased that you have chosen to read this book and, for a short while, walk along with me on this unique pathway to healing.

Reiki blessings,

Phylameana lila Désy

The EVERYTHING® Series

Editorial

Publishing Director	Gary M. Krebs
Managing Editor	Kate McBride
Copy Chief	Laura MacLaughlin
Acquisitions Editor	Eric M. Hall
Development Editor	Julie Gutin
Production Editor	Jamie Wielgus

Production

Production Director	Susan Beale
Production Manager	Michelle Roy Kelly
Series Designers	Daria Perreault
	Colleen Cunningham
Cover Design	Paul Beatrice
	Frank Rivera
Layout and Graphics	Colleen Cunningham
	Rachael Eiben
	Michelle Roy Kelly
	John Paulhus
	Daria Perreault
	Erin Ring
Series Cover Artist	Barry Littmann
Interior Digital Illustrator	Norma Medley

Visit the entire Everything® Series at everything.com

THE
EVERYTHING®
REIKI
BOOK

Channel your positive energy to
reduce stress, promote healing, and
enhance your quality of life

Phylameana lila Désy

Adams Media
Avon, Massachusetts

To my husband, sons, and daughter

An Everything® Series Book.
Everything® and everything.com® are registered trademarks of F+W Publications, Inc.

Published by Adams Media, an F+W Publications Company
57 Littlefield Street, Avon, MA 02322 U.S.A.
www.adamsmedia.com
ISBN 10: 1-59337-030-X
ISBN 13: 978-1-59337-030-5
Printed in the United States of America.

J I H G F E D

Library of Congress Cataloging-in-Publication Data
Désy, Phylameana lila.
The everything reiki book / Phylameana lila Désy.
p.   cm.
(An everything series book)
ISBN 1-59337-030-X
1. Reiki (Healing system) I. Title. II. Series: Everything series.

RZ403.R45D79 2004
615.8'51–dc22

2003019607

This publication is designed to provide accurate and authoritative information with regard to the subject matter covered. It is sold with the understanding that the publisher is not engaged in rendering legal, accounting, or other professional advice. If legal advice or other expert assistance is required, the services of a competent professional person should be sought.
　　—From a *Declaration of Principles* jointly adopted by a Committee of the American Bar Association and a Committee of Publishers and Associations

Many of the designations used by manufacturers and sellers to distinguish their products are claimed as trademarks. Where those designations appear in this book and Adams Media was aware of a trademark claim, the designations have been printed with initial capital letters.

This book is available at quantity discounts for bulk purchases.
For information, call 1-800-289-0963.

Contents

Acknowledgments

Reiki hugs and love, as well as my most heartfelt gratitude, go to all my friends and family members who provided me with the love, support, and encouragement I needed to undertake the writing of this book. This includes, but is not exclusive to, Amber M. Keith, Jonni K. Hecker, Morgan E. Wagner, Derric N. Wagner, the Reverend Beverley J. Voss, Mary J. Shomon, Norma J. Todd, and Linda S. Meyer. A very special thanks to my partner in life and sweetheart, Joe Désy, for his patience and sensible advice that helped me produce the final manuscript for the publisher.

Top Ten Benefits of
Practicing Reiki

1. Reiki is an effective self-help tool that promotes balance, relaxation, and overall well-being.

2. Reiki serves as an immediate first-aid response during times of trauma and injury.

3. Reiki is a community in which its practitioners automatically become members of its energetically connected family.

4. Reiki harms no one and serves as a complementary tool for assisting all other types of healing therapies.

5. Reiki helps practitioners develop stronger and healthier relationships with their loved ones.

6. Reiki helps practitioners bond spiritually with their environment.

7. Reiki extends its healing properties into all past, present, and future experiences that need soothing.

8. Reiki brings awareness, allowing practitioners to bring to light any innate intuitive abilities that have been buried or repressed.

9. Reiki's restorative properties are especially helpful in the care that follows medical treatments or surgical procedures.

10. Our pets benefit from Reiki energies by becoming healthier and calmer under a practitioner's care.

Introduction

▶USUI REIKI IS A SIMPLE and natural system of touch healing that originated in Japan through the discovery of a Zen Buddhist named Mikao Usui. The history and healing techniques used in Reiki are continuously passed down from teacher to student through a unique attunement process. Today, there are a variety of different lineages, all of which stem from this one man's influence.

Although Reiki is a spiritual healing art, it is not associated with any one belief system or doctrine, organized or otherwise. For this reason, Reiki practitioners make up a very diverse community. Reiki can be practiced by anyone who is open to its love energies. All that you need to give yourself a Reiki treatment are your hands, your body, and a willingness to touch it. Regardless of the status of your health, whether you are as fit as a fiddle or troubled by dis-ease or injury, Reiki can offer great benefits. When you are ill, Reiki treatments can help restore you to good health. When you are healthy, Reiki treatments will reinforce your vitality and strengthen your immune system.

Reiki is a holistic healing modality that encourages relaxation and relieves suffering. Its gentle action makes it a perfect instrument to have readily available under all circumstances. As you learn and begin to use Reiki, you will discover that it is easily accessible in any situation because it "turns on" automatically whenever you place your hands either on your body or on another person's body.

Extremely adaptable, Reiki complements other types of health treatments. Preop and postop Reiki treatments will often shorten the care period following surgery because Reiki accelerates the healing process. Also, Reiki treatments can easily be conducted in your home because no special equipment is required. The recipient can relax in a bed or recliner during the Reiki session. It would be wonderful if all households had at least one member in their family who practices Reiki, and this could very well happen in a few short years, as long as the use of Reiki continues to spread as quickly as it has in the past fifteen years.

The information in this book was written from the perspective of an Usui Reiki practitioner who was initially trained in Usui Shiki Ryoho, the traditional Reiki system primarily taught in the Western hemisphere.

However, there are many different Reiki systems that have emerged since the early 1980s. All of these newer Reiki systems have branched out from the Usui Reiki lineage. Many of these newer systems and their various similarities and differences are reviewed in Chapter 19. In this book's final chapter, you will also find information about other related touch therapies.

The Everything® Reiki Book is meant to present Reiki not only as a healing art, but also as a way of life. Reiki is so simple that Reiki Level I, the first of three levels of training, can be learned in only a few short hours. And yet, after a person takes that first-level Reiki class and becomes attuned to Reiki, he or she will be changed forever. The changes that may occur will vary from person to person, but these are changes that will ultimately be positive.

Balance comes to both the giver and receiver of Reiki's *ki* energies. In this book, the term *practitioner* is used to represent the person giving a Reiki treatment. The term *recipient* represents the person receiving it. Everyone who has been attuned to any level of Reiki may be called a "Reiki practitioner."

Reading about Reiki can be helpful in learning the basics. However, merely reading about it is not enough for anyone who truly desires to know what Reiki is all about. The healing art of Reiki needs to be experienced personally in order to fully nourish one's mind, body, and spirit, and it is only in this way that a person can arrive at a complete understanding of Reiki. Ⓔ

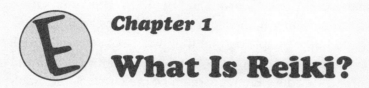

Chapter 1

What Is Reiki?

Usui Reiki Ryoho is an ancient hands-on healing art that intentionally channels ki energies to promote balance and well-being. The term *Reiki* is derived from two Japanese syllables, *rei* and *ki* (pronounced "ray key"), meaning Universal Life Energy. *Rei* represents the source of this energy and *ki* represents the energy's movement within and around us.

Reiki Is Energy

Reiki is the source of Universal Life Energy, and it is also a term used to describe the healing modality that accesses and transmits that energy. Reiki as a healing instrument operates through the concept that there is an unlimited supply of Universal Life Energy available for us to tap into.

Some believe that the Universal Life Energy, or Reiki, first emerged through the Creator. Many names can be traced back to this source, the diversity of these names implying that they were conceived through the auspices of different belief systems. Among these names are Universal Life Force, God-power, Goddess Energy, Breath of the Great Spirit, Nature, and Divinity.

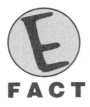

Ki is the Japanese term that refers to the life force, or living energy, that connects us to everything and sustains our life breath. The Chinese refer to this force as *chi,* or *qi,* the Hindus know it as *prana,* the Greeks as *pneuma,* the Polynesians as *mana,* and the Egyptians as *ka.*

It can be difficult to describe what Reiki is to someone who has not come into contact with it. How would you describe the wind to someone who had never experienced it? We cannot actually see the wind. We can feel and see only the effects of the wind; we feel its warmth or coolness against our skin when a breeze is gentle, and we see its strength when trees and homes are leveled during hurricanes. Wind upsets our hair, sweeps and scatters leaves about, waves our flags, and so on. It is an external force that we feel outside of our bodies. In contrast, Reiki could conceivably be compared to wind internalized. Reiki's life source fluctuates within our bodies.

How Reiki Enters the Body

There are different opinions about how Reiki enters the body. Some people believe it is pulled upward from the earth's grounding energies through the soles of the feet. Others believe it enters from a celestial source through the top of the head at the crown. Others feel it enters through the *tan tien,* or root chakra. Plausibly, it is a combination of all of these.

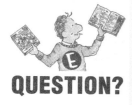

QUESTION?

What is the *tan tien*?
The *tan tien* (pronounced "dawn tea in") is located approximately 2.5 inches below the navel and about 2 inches inward. You can access this area by pushing both your index fingers and middle fingers into this soft tummy area. The *tan tien* is considered to be the center of our ki, where truth and inner knowledge reside. In martial arts, this center is used to draw upon power.

How Reiki Flows from the Body

In applying Reiki to the recipient, healing energies flow out of the practitioner's body through the palms of the hands as they touch the recipient's body. The flow varies in speed, depending on various factors such as the extent of the recipient's illness, degree of blockage, his or her readiness to accept change, and so on. The source offers an unlimited supply of Reiki so that we, as facilitators of Reiki, are never depleted. You can learn more about giving Reiki to others in Chapter 7.

Profound and Yet So Simple

Reiki, in its purest form, is an uncomplicated system of healing. You do not have to believe in Reiki for it to work. The facilitator cannot claim or take responsibility for healing or nonhealing when Reiki is applied. Reiki works at the level of acceptance of the person who is receiving it. Acceptance is not a matter of faith or belief. Acceptance suggests that there is a willingness to move from a painful experience into a less painful experience.

How Does Reiki Work?

The question of how Reiki works often arises among those who are newly exposed to Reiki. Actually, most people will take one of three primary approaches in questioning the workings of Reiki:

1. **Close-minded skepticism.** Naturally, there will always be skeptics who look for answers as to how Reiki works—or question whether it works at all. Unfortunately, the individuals who desire to dissect and scrutinize Reiki before ever trying it often overlook the simplicity of Reiki's profound gift.

2. **Openhearted acceptance.** Free-spirited individuals will jump right in with a willingness to take Reiki at face value, seldom questioning why or how it works. They are focused on results and are not overly concerned about the workings of Reiki. This casual ideology is certainly okay, since Reiki harms no one and does not interfere with other health treatments.

3. **Open-minded curiosity.** A third group looking at Reiki may be described as open-minded individuals with a profound curiosity and a healthy dose of skepticism. This diverse group is genuinely interested in learning more about Reiki.

In truth, nobody knows exactly how or why Reiki works. While it is clear that it does work, modern science has, at the present time, provided no reasonable explanation for it.

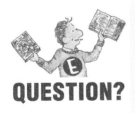

QUESTION?

Is Reiki a religion?
No. Having a belief system is not necessary for Reiki to work. Reiki does not infringe on your right to believe what you wish and does not require you to change or switch your religious faith. Christians, pagans, agnostics, Hindus, Buddhists, and Jews may freely adopt Reiki as a means to heal and bring harmony into their lives.

Story: Ticktock

A woman was walking along the business district on her way to meet a friend for lunch at a local restaurant. Earlier, she had taken a wrong turn and had lost her way. After she got her bearings and was once again on a familiar street, she wondered how much time she had lost and if she would be late for her luncheon.

She remembered that there was an antique-clock shop on the next block, so she decided she would go in and find out what time it was. When she stepped inside, she saw hundreds of clocks displaying different times. Sitting in the corner at a desk was an older gentleman, a clock maker, hunched over some watch parts he was toiling with. He looked up and asked the woman if he could help her.

She answered, "Oh yes please, I'd like to know about the time."

Thinking that someone was interested in the work he had spent his whole life laboring on, he enthusiastically began to show her all the minute parts and inner workings of a wristwatch he was in the process of assembling. He explained in great detail how everything works to make a timepiece.

The woman tried her best to show interest in the information that the man was sharing because she did not want to dampen his enthusiasm. But she really only wanted to know the time; it mattered little to her how a clock works.

The Reiki Analogy

This story demonstrates how we depend on our wall clocks and wristwatches to tell us the time. Seldom, if ever, are we concerned about the inner workings of the gadget that guides us though the hours and minutes of each day. Once you have experienced Reiki and have had positive results with it, the need to know why or how it works doesn't seem as important. This is not to say that further exploration of Reiki is not important. It's just that once you experience it, you'll know that it *does* work, and knowing how becomes less important.

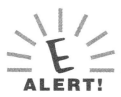

Reiki is not a gadget, and the way it works is actually less complicated than clockworks. No one had to invent it. Reiki has always been readily available and easily accessible to anyone.

The Power of Love Energy

Because of its gentle nature, Reiki is often described as a love energy. Its infinite healing power is limited only by our self-made boundaries. If you will allow it, Reiki will offer unconditional love to the inner child within you. As you open up to Reiki's love energies, you will discover the myriad of benefits it offers, including the following:

- Reiki replenishes vitality of life.
- It treats causes and symptoms of dis-eases.
- It clears away toxic and stagnant energies.
- It serves as a stress reliever and calming agent.
- It boosts the immune system.
- It enhances intuition.
- It does not conflict or interfere with any religious beliefs.
- It complements other healing modalities.
- It is always available, wherever you are.
- It promotes balance in all aspects of your life.
- It offers unconditional love.

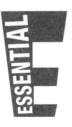

Many people in the healing community now substitute the term *dis-ease* for the word *disease*. In this way the emphasis is placed on the natural state of "ease" being imbalanced, or disrupted, with less focus on any particular ailment.

Channeling the Ki

Reiki is taught through the process of passing attunements from Master to student. Attuned Reiki students are then able to serve as conduits of an unlimited supply of Universal Life Energy that can be transferred to others, assisting them in healing.

Before attempting to draw upon this powerful healing reservoir, a person must be able to accommodate it, so that the life force can flow freely. Through the attunement process, a passageway is cleared within the body to serve as an empty vessel for channeling the ki energies.

Ki animates the body and gives life its pulse. Every living thing exists because of ki. Without ki, there is no life. When a person, animal, tree, or any living thing is in poor health, it is an indication that ki is not functioning as well as it could be. A sickly body is filled with toxins or blocked in some way, meaning that ki is not able to flow freely. The Reiki practitioner assists the recipient by channeling ki energies into the body to help break through blockages and flush out harmful toxins.

Experiencing Reiki

The best way to understand and appreciate Reiki is to experience it by having a full-body treatment. Reiki is for everyone and it is available to anyone who wants it. Moreover, you do not have to be attuned to Reiki in order to receive a treatment by a practitioner. All you need to do is locate a practitioner in your region and be willing to give Reiki a try.

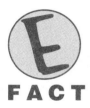

FACT

Complimentary minisessions are sometimes offered by Reiki practitioners in free workshops or drop-in clinics as a way to raise public awareness of Reiki. Also, some practitioners will offer free first-time full Reiki treatments to new customers in an attempt to increase their client base.

Much of this book focuses on becoming a Reiki practitioner, how to do self-Reiki, and how to go about giving Reiki treatments to family members or friends. But before you immerse yourself too deeply in the academic aspects of Reiki, and before signing up for a class and becoming attuned to Reiki, schedule a session for yourself with a practitioner and experience it firsthand. Reiki is for everyone, but not everyone is for Reiki. Consider getting at least one or two treatments before agreeing to an attunement.

Consider Attunements Carefully

Surprisingly, many people take a weekend Reiki class and become attuned to Reiki before ever having experienced a treatment or understanding that the attunement process is one of initiation and may act as a catalyst for life changes. Changes begin to take place as soon as Reiki is introduced into the body and begins its balancing process.

An attunement awakens the Reiki that is buried deeply inside your body. Once that awakening occurs, you will have committed yourself to changes in your life. Reiki flows constantly. It is always there and never goes away. Awareness of the possibility of experiencing subtle and, at other times, pronounced changes in your life as an aftereffect of an attunement can benefit you in the long run. You can learn more about the Reiki attunement process in Chapter 4.

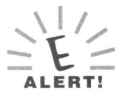
ALERT!

Reiki cannot ever cause you any harm. Rather, it works to bring about positive changes. However, since Reiki can also offer challenges while any change is occurring, it is better to postpone your attunement until you're fully prepared to handle the possible changes.

It is recommended that you interview the Reiki instructor before registering for your attunement class, and be sure to ask any questions pertinent to the attunement process. Some Reiki teachers give only one attunement to their students, whereas others give two or even four attunements.

Honoring the Reiki Rite

This book is not meant to serve as a substitute for taking a Reiki class. It is offered as an introduction to Reiki and should be used as a handbook in addition to taking classes. In order to practice Reiki, there is an initiation process that will open you up to Reiki. Becoming a Reiki practitioner is not something you can do on your own through reading a how-to book or watching an instructional video. Receiving Reiki training can be achieved in a one-day or two-day workshop, making access to it relatively effortless.

This is not to say that a person cannot tap into the life force and do energy-healing work without being attuned to Reiki. There are other energy-healing modalities, such as Pranic Healing and Healing Touch, which do not involve attunements. However, it is the initiation process involving attunements that makes Reiki different from other energy-healing techniques.

There are no substitutes for receiving Reiki attunements. Reading about Reiki is not a shortcut for taking a class. Some people have proclaimed themselves to be Reiki practitioners without ever having been attuned by a teacher. This is not ethical behavior and dishonors the Reiki Rite of Passage.

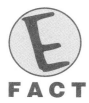

FACT

Reiki's roots can be traced to Japan through the work of Mikao Usui, the founder of the Usui System of Natural Healing. Hawayo Takata, a Japanese-American woman, introduced the teachings of Reiki to the United States. Since then, Reiki has spread to virtually every continent.

ABC's of Reiki

As you begin your acquaintance with Reiki, there are several keywords that can help you along the way. Use the following ABC list as an easy guide to learn what Reiki is and what Reiki can do. In the back of this book you will find an extensive glossary of Reiki terms with more detailed descriptions (see Appendix B).

- **Always available**—Reiki offers an unlimited supply of healing energies that are always available for us to draw upon.
- **Attunements**—Reiki is passed down from teacher to student through an initiation ritual that involves attunements.
- **Aura**—At the end of a Reiki session, Reiki practitioners sweep the person's aura. This is done to clear away any debris or negative energies that have surfaced from the physical body.
- **Balance**—Anytime Reiki is applied it goes about its work to bring balance to any imbalances.
- **Comfort**—Reiki's warm and gentle action soothes and comforts.

- **Complementary treatment**—Reiki complements and often increases the effectiveness of other treatments.
- **Distant healing**—Reiki treatments can be applied to recipients who are not in the same room as the practitioner.
- **Easing of physical and mental dis-ease**—Reiki's healing vibrations ease our physical dis-eases and handle conflicts in our mental states, as well as dysfunctions in the emotional and spiritual sides of our physical beings.
- **Enlightenment**—Reiki is a spiritual path that leads to enlightenment.
- **Flow**—Reiki flows automatically from one person to another through the palms of the hands.
- **Gassho**—Meditation prayer ritual that is often performed by the practitioner before and after a full-body Reiki treatment.
- **Guides**—Some Reiki practitioners have acknowledged having spiritual guides that assist them in their healing work.
- **Hand placements**—There are a dozen or so hand positions used in applying Reiki to cover the whole body.
- **Hayashi**—Retired naval officer Dr. Chujiro Hayashi was initiated as a Reiki Master by Mikao Usui.
- **Infinity**—Reiki's unlimited power offers an infinite number of ways to heal.
- **Intelligence**—Reiki is called "intelligent energy" because it works without focused intent, does not require our belief, and knows where it is most needed.
- **Japan**—Reiki's roots can be traced back to Japan, where Dr. Mikao Usui first learned of its power of healing.
- **Kanji**—Modified Chinese characters used in Japanese writing system; Reiki symbols are derived from kanji.
- **Ki**—The life force that flows through every living thing: humans, animals, plants, etc.
- **Love**—Reiki is known as "love energy" because of the warmth and feelings of care that it evokes.
- **Mt. Kurama**—Dr. Mikao Usui was awakened to the healing energies of Reiki after a twenty-one-day meditation fast on Mt. Kurama in Japan.
- **Meditation**—As Reiki energies are absorbed into the recipient's body, he or she will often be lulled into a relaxed and meditative state.

- **No harm**—Reiki is a completely safe, holistic, and natural way of treating dis-ease.
- **Nourishment**—Reiki is as nourishing to the body as air, food, and water.
- **Open heart**—Reiki's love energy opens our hearts.
- **Practitioner**—All levels of Reiki initiates are considered practitioners since they *practice* Reiki. Some, but not all, practitioners serve as healers in a clinical setting.
- **Prayer**—Reiki is very similar to prayer since the primary intent in applying Reiki is to request healing.
- **Qi (chi)**—The Chinese share the idea of ki, an energy that is present in all living things and in the universe.
- **Reiju**—The empowerment process used by Dr. Mikao Usui to pass Reiki to his students.
- **Sensei**—The Japanese title for "teacher."
- **Shares**—Reiki practitioners may meet in group settings, called Reiki shares, to practice Reiki among themselves.
- **Spirituality**—Although it is not a religion, Reiki has spiritual beginnings (it was discovered through meditation) and can lead to spiritual development with continued use.
- **Symbols**—Reiki incorporates the use of symbols in its attunement process, absentia sendings, and in hands-on treatments.
- **Touch therapy**—Reiki is a touch therapy that reinforces the inherent knowledge that we enjoy being touched.
- **Transformation**—Reiki is a transforming energy that brings about positive changes.
- **Unconditional love**—Reiki offers unconditional love to the inner child within us.
- **Universal Life Energy**—That is exactly what Reiki means.
- **Visualization**—Visualization techniques are employed in Reiki whenever the practitioner makes use of Reiki symbols.
- **Wisdom**—Reiki is wisdom.
- **Zoom**—Reiki energies hone in to wherever they are needed, regardless of where you place your hands.

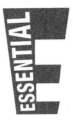

Laying on of the hands is a custom present in many cultures. In the New Testament of the Bible, you will find the following passage: "Do not neglect the gift that is in you, which was given to you by prophecy with the laying on of the hands of the eldership. Meditate on these things; give yourself entirely to them, that your progress may be evident to all" (1 Timothy 4:14–15).

The inclination to assist another person and provide comfort and reassurance when he or she is physically or emotionally hurt is an innate instinct in all of us. The principles of Reiki are based on this natural instinct. If you learn only one thing for certain about Reiki—that touching is healing—you will have embraced the heart of this ancient healing art. The rhythmic sensations brought about by Reiki's healing touch are the equivalent to its heartbeat.

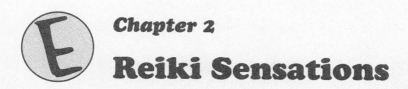

Chapter 2

Reiki Sensations

As Reiki energies flow between the practitioner and the recipient during the Reiki session, the two bodies may respond or react with particular sensations. Those sensations are nearly always pleasant. You may feel heat, warmth, cold, subtleness, steadfastness, or forcefulness. The fact that you can feel Reiki flowing, whether you are giving or receiving it, is verification that the energy is being welcomed.

What It Feels Like

Reiki works like a thermostat that regulates the body. Much like a furnace that automatically turns on and off to regulate the temperature, Reiki flows slowly or rapidly—as needed—to dispense balancing energies. Like a pendulum swinging back and forth, Reiki sometimes moves erratically, other times smoothly. These fluctuations of ki energy churning within us can often be felt as pins-and-needles tingling, hot flashes, goose bump chills, throbbing, etc.

During a Reiki treatment, both the Reiki practitioner and the recipient feel Reiki sensations. A practitioner's hands will often heat up as a result of the flow coursing through his palms. The recipient frequently feels sleepy and yawns repeatedly as incoming Reiki energies soothe and calm pent-up emotional tension and stress.

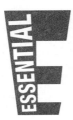

You may experience any of the following sensations during a Reiki session: heat or coolness, pins-and-needle tingling, vibrational buzzing, electrical sparks, numbness, throbbing, itchiness, and sleepiness.

Some people are more in tune with their bodies than others and will be able to share fantastic stories about feeling the different sensations that occur while using Reiki. They will talk about experiencing imagery, kinesthesia, and/or inner voices while either giving or receiving Reiki.

You May Not Feel Anything

Reiki sensations can be very subtle and may be overlooked, but with continued practice most people will begin to notice even the slightest shifts of energy. A few people will seldom, if ever, feel anything with Reiki beyond the tactile sensation of hands-to-body touch.

Fortunately, Reiki works whether you feel it or not. If you are having difficulty feeling sensations while giving a Reiki treatment, try closing your eyes. Keeping your eyes shut eliminates visual distractions, which will help you focus more on the person and the sensations.

Hot and Cold Hands

It is often taught that after receiving your Reiki Level I attunements you will develop hot hands. Having hot hands is supposedly a credible sign that the attunement worked and that you are now officially a channel for Reiki. Experiencing hot hands may very well indicate that Reiki has been awakened and you are now a genuine, functioning Reiki conduit. But if you do not experience hot hands, does that indicate nothing has happened and that your attunement was a failure? Not at all. Every person's attunement experience is unique. Being told that you need to experience hot hands or that your experience was somehow deficient because it was different from that of others is greatly misleading.

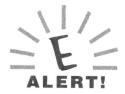

Always wash your hands with soap and water before applying Reiki. Avoid fragrant soaps and lotions, especially if the person you are treating may be allergic to the aromatic chemicals used in those products. If your hands are naturally cold, briskly rub your palms together for several seconds to warm them up before beginning treatment.

Temperature Variations

For some Reiki practitioners, hand temperature may change as they are giving Reiki treatments. These changes range from burning hot to icy cold. Sometimes, the practitioner's and the recipient's perception of the temperature will be different. For instance, as you are giving Reiki, you may feel that you're burning up, but your recipient may feel coolness from your touch. Or, it may be that you are experiencing cold hands, while the recipient may comment on the warmth of your hands.

Extrahealing Hands

Here is an experience that is not at all uncommon. Some Reiki recipients may feel that additional practitioners are participating in the Reiki session.

For instance, one woman reported that during a one-on-one session with the Reiki practitioner, she had felt two additional pairs of hands placed upon her body.

One explanation of the "extrahealing hands" sensation is that healing spirit guides are present. You can learn more in Chapter 11.

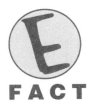

FACT

Maureen J. Kelly, author of *Reiki and the Healing Buddha*, says the sensations of the hands that Reiki practitioners experience can be explained by the Chinese philosophy of yin and yang. If the practitioner's hands are hot, it indicates the recipient's body has too much yang energy. If the hands are cold, the body has too much yin energy.

The Reiki Pulse

The pulsating sensation of Reiki can be felt in all parts of your body, but especially in the palms of your hands. This is because the palms are the outlets of Reiki energy. Reiki is like an anxious mother waiting at the door with open arms for her children to come home. Reiki wants to flow out of your hands and be put to good use. As soon as you place your hands on yourself, or someone else, Reiki automatically turns on.

After you are attuned to Reiki, you become a walking generator of sorts. Your body will heat up and start spewing out healing energies whenever you are near anyone who is receptive to Reiki. This feeling can overwhelm the newly attuned person, especially if he or she had not been advised beforehand that this could happen. Your immediate reaction may be to place your hands on the person, but this is not recommended. Never assume that you have the right to go up to a person and touch him or her just because your body's sensations are telling you that he or she is open to it. Always ask first.

You do not need to lay your hands on the person for Reiki to flow over to him or her. Simply put a smile on your face and allow Reiki to do all the transference; just being aware that you are a conduit for Reiki is sufficient. The receptive person doesn't need to be aware that anything is happening.

If you are among a crowd of people, such as sitting in a movie theater or shopping at the market, you probably won't be certain to whom the Reiki is actually flowing. Accept your role as a Reiki channel and try not to get caught up in a need-to-know mindset. It is not important to know where the Reiki is going. Simply let it flow. After a while, you won't even pay attention when Reiki is flowing from you because it will become a routine occurrence.

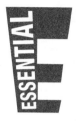

Healers who are familiar with the healing properties of gemstones will sometimes combine the healing energies of specific crystals in their Reiki sessions with clients. Metals, on the other hand, are conductors of energy and will absorb Reiki, cheating the receiver of the full benefit. Magnetic jewelry also presents a problem, as it polarizes the Reiki energy.

Balls of Pulsating Energy

There may be times when Reiki will ball up in your hands, creating a circling orb of energy. Imagine having a tennis ball glued to the palm of your hand. No matter how hard you try, you cannot shake it off. Now, imagine that this tennis ball is a living organism that has a pulse.

Experiencing these pulsating balls of energy in your hands can be an odd or even disturbing sensation, but there is nothing to worry about. Reiki isn't flowing anywhere outside of you, because there is no specific place for it to go. However, this may very well be an indication that self-Reiki is needed. Take advantage of this excess of energy in your hands and place your hands on your body. Allowing the Reiki to flow into your body should help reduce or release the ball of energy from your palms.

Anytime you feel an excess of energy building up in your body, you can take advantage of this by infusing inanimate objects with Reiki. Placing Reiki inside objects transforms them into healing instruments. Reiki can be put into any object by holding the object between your hands and allowing Reiki energies to pour into it. Reiki Level II practitioners can also place Reiki symbols, along with their energies, into these objects, making them become even more powerful. Any of the following objects may be filled with Reiki:

- Reiki your bed pillow, filling it with Reiki energies for a restful night's sleep.
- Reiki your bath water—nothing feels more soothing than soaking in a Reiki bath.
- Reiki your lamps and light bulbs—their illuminations will have a Reiki glow!
- Reiki your aromatherapy candles, incense sticks, and flower essences.
- Reiki your shampoo, skin lotions, and toothpaste.
- Reiki your vitamins and prescription medications.
- Reiki your shoes—this will be a special treat for your feet.
- Reiki your computer to reduce the number of system crashes.
- Reiki your telephone to help you be more patient with disruptive callers.

Vibrating Hands

Water pipes expand and contract to accommodate the water as it flows through them. In this same manner your body also adjusts to the flow of Reiki being channeled through your body. When Reiki is being drawn out of your palms at a faster rate or in larger proportions than you are accustomed to, you may experience your hands vibrating. The vibration occurs as a result of the Reiki gushing through your body so quickly that it gets backed up into your hands. Reiki is trying to get out and go where it needs to go, but the openings in your palms are too narrow to pass it on efficiently.

This is not an insurmountable problem. You've done nothing wrong, so there is no need to be overly concerned. Aside from being uncomfortable, the shakiness in your hands is merely signifying that the person receiving Reiki from you is in great need. The recipient is sponging up Reiki as fast as he or she can get it.

Other Sensations

Aside from the vibrational sensation in your hands, you may also experience soreness in your wrists and the joints of your fingers. In treating people with severe illnesses, you may feel a powerful pulling of Reiki energies from your neck, shoulders, and down your arms as well. If you find channeling greater volumes of Reiki painful or uncomfortable when treating someone, remove your hands from the recipient from time to time to give your hands a chance to rest. You can alternate—ten minutes hands on, ten minutes hands off, and so on.

Facilitating the Flow

Reiki flows in the direction of the easiest pathway. When the natural course of a river comes up against a dam, the water pools up in that area until it either breaks through the blockade or reroutes itself by traveling around the obstacle, moving through to the next available open channel.

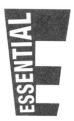

Reiki is just like a river. Its energies flow through our bodies, following the most natural path in filling us up. The hand placements used to administer Reiki allow the energy to enter the body through different channels.

There are twelve basic hand placements that are used in giving a full-body Reiki treatment—four placements on the head, four on the front of the body, and four placements on the back of the body. Applying Reiki for five minutes in each of these placements helps to distribute Reiki evenly over the whole body. However, when hands are placed on one area, sometimes the person will experience hot spots elsewhere. For example, you may have your hands placed on the person's throat, yet the person will feel a trickling of energy running down one or both of her legs. Always know that Reiki goes where it needs to go.

Dealing with Blockages

As you move your hands through the various hand placements, you may come to a position on the body that feels blocked. When you no longer feel Reiki flowing from your palms, your first impulse may be to move on to the next hand placement—but hold on. Blocked areas are denser and often need more attention given to them. Sometimes all you will need to do is shift your hands an inch or two from that position, either up or down, in order to get Reiki to start flowing again. If this doesn't work, be patient. Keep your hands on the recipient's body where you sense Reiki is being blocked for a full five minutes before moving along.

In Tune with Your Etheric Hand

No pressure is to be applied to the body when giving Reiki. Place your hands gently on the body. However, there may be situations when your hands might feel as if they are actually sinking deeply into the body while giving Reiki. This sinking or magnetic pulling sensation happens when your etheric hand extends itself into the deep tissues.

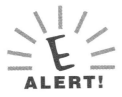

During a Reiki treatment, you may sense a waft of fragrance. This can be an indication that a spirit guide, angelic being, or Ascended Master is visiting your session. Some Reiki practitioners have reported sensing Mrs. Hawayo Takata's presence through a subtle floral fragrance.

Removing your physical hand before your etheric hand has retracted itself to join the physical hand can cause a disruption in the healing session. If your hands feel like they are stuck to the body, it is likely that this kind of deeper etheric healing is occurring. It is advantageous to keep your hands in position for an extended period while this deeper healing work is being done. If it is not feasible for you to keep your hands in position due to time constraints or some other unavoidable reason, be sure to remove your hands slowly without any abrupt movements. Take care to be as gentle as possible.

A Vessel That Never Empties

When you are giving a Reiki treatment to someone, you are giving your time and your intent to assist; you are not giving away any of your own energy. Reiki is in infinite supply. It never runs out. As a Reiki practitioner you are making yourself available as a vessel through which Reiki can be accessed.

During and after giving a Reiki treatment, you may feel a variety of emotions. These feelings can run the gamut from exhaustion to exhilaration, or something in between. However, these feelings have not occurred because you have been drained of energy. Something else is going on. It is possible that you were in great need of Reiki yourself and, by giving Reiki to another person, you also received Reiki. Reiki will always attend to the practitioner's needs as well as the recipient's. Reiki always offers a double treatment. If you routinely feel tired after giving Reiki to someone else, this is an indication that you need to focus on self-treatments for a while. After attending to your own needs, you will feel better and more capable of sharing Reiki with others.

Feeling the Pain of Others

If a practitioner is empathic, touching other people may cause her to develop mirrored illnesses. However, having empathic abilities is not a requirement of Reiki, nor does it enhance Reiki's effectiveness. Empaths need to learn that the ability to "take on" or "feel" another person's pain or emotions is best used as a diagnostic tool. Don't hold on to the empathetic feelings—they must be released as soon as possible.

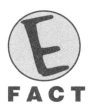

FACT

People with empathic natures are also known as highly sensitive people, ultrasensitive people, or people with "overexcitabilities." According to the research of Jim and Amy Hallowes ("lay experts" on the subject whose research results appear on their Web site, HighlySensitivePeople.com), highly sensitive people, or HSP, make up 15 to 20 percent of the world's population.

When you find yourself feeling the sensations of someone else's emotions or pains within your own body, take some gentle, deep breaths and ask the person you are treating to take a few deep breaths as well. This should help break up the blocked energy so that you can continue the treatment without continued discomfort. You can learn more about empathic healers in Chapter 11.

Perception Techniques

Reiji Ho and Byosen Reikan Ho are two Reiki techniques taught in Japan. These techniques focus the practitioner on perceiving sensations within the body of the person being treated. You can learn how to develop your intuitive abilities and use intent when treating illness and imbalance. The learning process is gradual, as you continue to practice giving Reiki treatments to others.

Byosen Reikan Ho

Byosen Reikan Ho is a scanning technique that is done before and after a Reiki session. The practitioner's hands are moved over the body, without touching the person, to detect dis-eases and imbalances. This technique can be used to detect and treat dis-ease that has not yet manifested in the body. It is also used to treat residual toxins from past illnesses as a preventative measure against reoccurrence. Byosen Reikan Ho is not a diagnostic procedure, but a technique performed to locate and treat illness.

Reiji Ho

Reiji Ho is the intuitive ability to know where imbalances are in the body without touching it. The practitioner's hands are intuitively led to areas and specific spots on which to lay his or her hands in order to facilitate a healing. This is the technique that was taught before the Reiki hand placements were developed. ⒺⒽ

Chapter 3

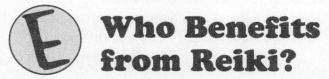

Who Benefits from Reiki?

Reiki helps to restore and strengthen each person's life force. No matter what the individual's need is, Reiki will support his or her stability and well-being. Reiki does not discriminate. Its availability is constant. Treatment can be received by anyone, anywhere, anytime. The list of benefits that Reiki offers to its recipients is extensive. Any person, animal, or plant that is in need can be helped with Reiki treatments, given either through the laying on of hands or through distant healing.

Reiki During Pregnancy

Reiki can be beneficial for all age groups, even for those who are not yet born. Pregnant women who are attuned to Reiki can extend love to their unborn children by laying their hands on their belly and allowing Reiki energies to be taken in by their babies.

Some Reiki practitioners feel that if a woman is attuned to Reiki during her pregnancy, her baby is also attuned to the energies. What a wonderful gift to offer your child before his or her birthday!

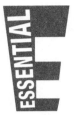

It is perfectly safe for a pregnant woman to have a full-body Reiki treatment. Reiki will flow to both mother and child. What a bargain, getting two treatments for the price of one!

For Young Children

Reiki's gentle and noninvasive nature is also perfect for treating the ills and upsets of young children. Children are extremely receptive to Reiki's positive effects and will normally welcome it without any apprehension, especially when they receive Reiki treatments from their parents.

Reiki treatments are to be given to children much in the same manner as they are given to adults. The basic hand placements are the same. However, the treatment will not last as long. Reiki energies travel swiftly through a child's body—unlike adults, children don't yet have years of accumulated toxins or blockages that tend to slow down the treatment process. If the child becomes restless or fidgety when receiving Reiki, the treatment should be ended. Children will often instinctively sit up and move away from the Reiki practitioner when they feel they have had enough.

Attuning Children

Babies and toddlers can be attuned to Reiki, but they are not mature enough to learn how to practice it. Children younger than five years of age lack the comprehension skills to understand the concepts of Reiki.

Most children between the ages of five and twelve have the ability to learn Reiki and can be attuned to the first level. One or two Reiki attunements may be all that are needed to attune children to Reiki Level I (traditionally, four attunements are required for adults). Also, young children should not be expected to sit through a full day or even a half day of Reiki instruction, since their attention spans are meager. Teachers should attune the child and give him or her only basic instructions. Afterward, it is appropriate for the parent to carefully guide and assist the child in the use of Reiki in the home. For this reason, the only children who should be attuned to Reiki are those with a parent or other adult in the home who is an experienced practitioner of Reiki.

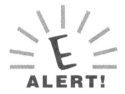

ALERT!

Children should be cautioned not to force their Reiki hands upon classmates who may not understand or appreciate what they are attempting to do. Instead, have them focus on practicing Reiki at home. It is essential that your child be ready for Reiki. Children enjoy giving Reiki to their dolls and stuffed animals, as well as to their pets and siblings.

If you are considering having your child attuned, it is a good idea to arrange a time for the child and teacher to meet with each other before the day of attunement arrives. Preferably, this meeting would take place in the same environment where the class would be held. Look to see that your child is comfortable and at ease with both the teacher and the environment. If you notice that your child shows fear or appears resistant in any way, you should hold off on scheduling a class. It is essential that your child be ready for Reiki.

It's Good for Seniors

Reiki is suitable for people of all ages. But because of Reiki's pain management capabilities, seniors especially welcome it—probably because it offers help in alleviating the aches and pains associated with aging.

Reiki's effectiveness varies from person to person. Some ailments respond more favorably to Reiki than others. Also, some people are more receptive to Reiki. It is theorized that both children and senior citizens, as specific age groups, are more receptive than middle-aged persons. Children are inherently more curious and trusting of the world at large. Just as they depend on their parents to feed, clothe, and take care of them, when it comes to accepting Reiki, they are naturally more amenable to the energies that are offered.

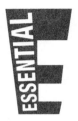

Alzheimer patients can be attuned to Reiki. Although they may not understand or remember the attunement, their caregivers can remind them each day to place their hands on their bodies. They will reap the benefits of Reiki energies flowing into their bodies whenever they touch themselves.

As children grow into adolescents and young adults, they become less dependent on their caregivers. Children anticipate the time when they will be able to make their own decisions and escape from being under the full authority of their guardians. The increasing maturity that accompanies children into their late teens and early adulthood years instills in them the desire to spread their wings and become strong and capable individuals. They become willing and satisfied to take care of themselves, no longer under the ever-watchful eyes of their parents. If an illness or accident occurs after attaining a strong sense of self-sufficiency, they often become reluctant to accept assistance for fear of losing their newly found independence.

Far too many young adults, as well as those in their middle years, will stubbornly take a determined stance, declaring "I can do it for myself" or "I don't need any help." Fear of losing independence is often the reason why some people don't seek out professional medical assistance until they have become very sick. They will stubbornly refuse to ask for help until their discomforts have progressively worsened and they feel incapable of self-care. Unfortunately, this reluctance to accept assistance from others can also effectively block Reiki from flowing optimally.

Many seniors, on the other hand, have come to the realization that they can no longer do everything for themselves. They have also learned that life can be easier if they stop resisting help when and where it is offered. Because of their diminished physical or mental capabilities, many seniors have been forced to depend on others in order for their needs to be met. As a result, seniors are normally more readily accepting of Reiki's assistance. See Chapter 7 for basic hand placements for performing Reiki on seniors.

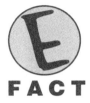

FACT

Energy medicine (Healing Touch, Therapeutic Touch, and Reiki) is today becoming recognized as both a beneficial and complementary therapy to conventional medicine as well as an alternative treatment especially helpful in pain management.

A Caregiving Practice

The caregivers in our medical communities include doctors, chiropractors, nurses, counselors, therapists, nursing home aides, and hospice workers. However, the title of caregiver also applies to individuals who personally assist their relatives and friends who are aged, ailing, or indisposed. Parents are caregivers as well—they provide care for their kids. All Reiki practitioners are caregivers in the sense that they give of themselves when caring for others with Reiki treatments.

Caregivers are at high risk of physical and emotional burnout. Taking care of another person, especially if his or her needs are considerable, can result in a great expenditure of one's physical and emotional energy. Therefore, it is vital that the caregiver's depleted energies are replenished. Fortunately, caregivers can rely on Reiki not only by giving treatments to their charges, but also by carrying out self-treatments to keep themselves energized and balanced.

Reiki and Pets

Many people today look for a holistic approach to treating illnesses in their animal companions. Touch therapies, such as Reiki, Tellington TTouch, and shiatsu, are frequently sought out to help bring relief to animals that are suffering. Other complementary therapies used in holistic pet care are homeopathy, aromatherapy, and flower essence therapy.

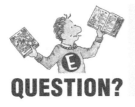

QUESTION?

What is Tellington TTouch?
Tellington TTouch is an animal touch therapy modality based on circular movements of the fingers and hands all over the body to accelerate the healing of injuries or ailments.

Animal lovers are sensitive to their pets' illnesses. Likewise, pets can be sensitive to the sufferings of their caregivers. Many dogs and cats absorb Reiki energies more quickly than humans. This could simply be the result of their size (at least for most cats and small- to medium-sized dog breeds), but more likely it is because they inherently understand what Reiki is. Most cats and dogs will accept the energies they need and allow you to place your hands on them freely. When they have had enough, they will simply walk away. A full treatment could be over in five minutes. Treatments seldom last more than twenty minutes.

You can give Reiki to your pets by touching, stroking, or patting them. Reiki can also be sent to animals through distant healing if they are skittish or confused by your touch—or if you are allergic to an animal's fur or dander. Distant healing is a must for treating nondomestic animals such as terrestrial wildlife, zoo animals, and aquatic creatures.

Here is how Reiki can help your pet:

- It accelerates the healing of physical injuries.
- It promotes peace and calmness.
- It treats trauma from accidents or surgery, nervousness, and fear.
- It reduces stress and suffering.
- It helps promote bonding between animal and pet owner.
- It treats behavioral problems: chewing, biting, scratching, excessive barking, and so on.
- It offers a comforting transitional energy when it is time for your pet to depart from this world.

Dealing with the Skeptics

Approaching new ideas with an ounce or two of healthy skepticism is always a good thing. Common sense provokes us to first scrutinize any new undertaking or belief system. We certainly don't feel good about our judgment when we fall victim to fantastic or miraculous claims that don't hold true in the end. It is simply good rational thinking to be cautious of anything being promoted as a "magic pill" or "cure-all remedy," and it makes perfect sense to be wary of outlandish claims that tout amazing results from using various health products and healing techniques.

However, some people don't question new ideas. They simply reject them out of hand. These people enjoy pointing out flawed notions and poking fun at idealist thinkers. Skeptics consider supporters and devotees of Reiki to be nothing more than a bunch of gullible individuals. Sadly, these people may never have the opportunity to appreciate how Reiki works because of their refusals to give it a try.

Reiki Responds Uniquely to Each Individual

Reiki does not discriminate when it comes to selecting who is deserving of treatment based on what he or she believes. Reiki treats imbalance. Because each person has his or her own specific imbalances, using Reiki will bring about a unique response in each person. This is why explaining how Reiki works to someone who has not experienced it can be so frustrating or difficult. One recipient will report that Reiki is a miraculous healing technique that cured her addiction to nicotine. Another recipient might say that, although his experience with Reiki was relaxing, it didn't offer a cure. A third recipient's account of Reiki, again based on her personal experiences, might be something entirely different.

There are many benefits derived from Reiki, but the results of treatments can vary as the result of several different factors:

- Did the recipient receive only one treatment, or did he or she have cumulative Reiki treatments?
- How advanced was the recipient's illness before Reiki treatments were applied?

- Is a particular imbalance or dis-ease offering a spiritual lesson to the recipient, a lesson that needs to be experienced rather than cured?
- Were the recipient's expectations too high, ultimately setting him or her up for failure?
- How receptive is the recipient to allowing Reiki into his or her body?

Belief and Receptivity

Believing in Reiki and being receptive to Reiki energies are two very different things. Reiki will work whether or not a person believes in it. However, if a person is not receptive to Reiki, consciously or unconsciously, its energies will have a tough time penetrating that barrier. This is why some people who truly believe that Reiki will work are disappointed when it appears to have no beneficial effect on them. On the other hand, the skeptics who do not believe Reiki will work may very well experience positive results with Reiki because their bodies are naturally receptive to Reiki's healing vibrations.

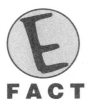

FACT

Reiki will treat numerous physical maladies, emotional imbalances, mental disturbances, and spiritual afflictions. Reiki will also extend its healing energies to nurture your environment and strengthen your relationships.

Reiki Benefits Everyone

Reiki's gift of increased energy and vitality can be extended to anyone. It doesn't matter what a person's gender, race, intelligence level, or financial status is. Reiki is not a healing energy reserved only for the elite, wealthy, educated, or spiritually evolved. Reiki is free to anyone who wants it. It does not cost anything but a little of your time.

Treating Root Causes

Because Reiki naturally flows to where it is needed, its natural course is to first deal with any apparent symptoms of illness or dis-ease. When

Reiki treatments are discontinued after your symptoms have diminished or been eliminated, don't be surprised if these conditions recur. Reiki will only serve as a Band-Aid if you abandon its use too hastily. Through consistent and continued use of Reiki, the root cause of any given illness can be treated. It is when the root cause is treated fully that Reiki can be called a "cure."

Benefits of Reiki

The list of benefits that Reiki offers is comprehensive. Basically, Reiki will benefit you by empowering you whenever you feel weakened or downtrodden. Here is a list of some of the specific benefits Reiki offers:

- Reiki's calming effects can reduce our anxieties and panicky behavior.
- It may go to the core of imbalances embedded within our bodies to bring about balance.
- Pain, stresses, and agitations that are associated with long-term suffering can benefit from cumulative Reiki treatments.
- Reiki can be safely used in conjunction with all other conventional health practices.
- Reiki offers the kind of energetic vitality that can spark our innate creativity.
- Reiki's ability to awaken and sharpen our psychic perceptions heightens awareness of our dreams.
- Blessing our foods and drinks with Reiki before consuming them will vitalize and purify them.
- Reiki's gentle energies are conducive to comforting anyone who is suffering from grief. It helps the grief process run its course in a calmer or less painful way.
- Reiki tames discord and trouble, bringing harmony to the recipient or situation that is out of sync.
- The swiftness of Reiki's healing properties has demonstrated that it is an effective first-aid treatment for injuries.
- Reiki will treat emotional wounds and memories that are hurting our inner child.

- Reiki assists us in letting go of the aspects within our lives that negatively impact us.
- The manifesting facets of Reiki help to bring our intentions and goals to fruition.
- Reiki can expedite the body's natural healing ability, reducing the recovery periods that follow surgeries and injuries.
- Reiki's relaxing energies can induce sleep and relieve insomnia.
- Using Reiki may awaken or improve spiritual awareness.
- Reiki releases toxins, clearing our bodies of impurities and stagnant energies.
- Reiki will penetrate beyond obvious systematic conditions of the body and treat the underlying causes of illness.
- Reiki can help you deal with special situations in your life such as exams, job interviews, divorce, career changes, and family illness.

This list could be expanded for several more pages; there is simply no limit to the benefits that Reiki can bestow on those who are receptive to it. All of us can benefit from it—and so can our children, our parents and grandparents, and our animal companions. Even skeptical-minded individuals who look cautiously at Reiki can benefit from Reiki if they are willing to explore its possibilities. For you to reap the full benefits that Reiki has to offer, simply sign up for a Reiki class. In as little as a few hours you will be certified as a Level I practitioner.

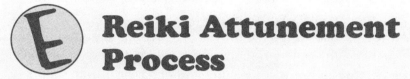

Chapter 4

Reiki Attunement Process

A Reiki attunement is an expansion process, or, you could say, a knock at the door that opens to a space that already exists. That "space" is a passageway within our bodies through which the Universal Life Energy travels. Receiving a Reiki attunement can be a meaningful or even a life-altering experience. The attunement ritual is performed with a Reiki Master/Teacher. Choosing the right person to initiate you into the world of Reiki can make all the difference in how you experience your Reiki attunement.

Choosing the Appropriate Reiki Master

The term *master* implies a person who possesses insightful knowledge and esteemed wisdom. Perhaps this is representative of some Reiki Masters. But most others are bumbling along in life the best way they can, just like everyone else, and don't wish to be regarded as having any special elite status or powers. Respect them, yes, but don't worship them! In Reiki, the title merely means "teacher."

As you probably remember from past school days, not all teachers are equal. Most people are much more willing to study with teachers whose personalities are compatible and don't clash with their students'. Moreover, people learn best when a teacher displays integrity and a passion for his or her subject.

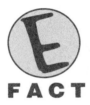

FACT

In Japan, Reiki attunements were originally called "empowerments." The term "attunement" appeared after Hawayo Takata brought Reiki to the United States. Other terms that have been used to describe attunement are *initiation, awakening, expansion,* and *transmission.*

Meeting Prospective Teachers

Interviewing Reiki Masters in order to find the appropriate person to initiate you into the world of Reiki can be almost as frustrating as shopping for the perfect pair of shoes. You may have to try on quite a few pairs of shoes before you find the perfect fit. Don't settle for penny loafers—even if they fit—when you really have your eye on those crimson leather pumps. Another customer may find the penny loafers quite comfy to wear, but they aren't for you. When choosing your Reiki teacher, take your time and consider your options carefully. The relationship between Reiki teacher and student is not one to take lightly.

The interview does not have to be a lengthy process. A three- to five-minute phone call should be a sufficient amount of time for you to get either a good or bad feeling about your prospective teacher.

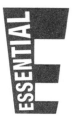

Don't expect a potential teacher to invest her time in discussions with you for more than around ten minutes before you have committed yourself to signing up for a class. If you wish to speak extensively with a teacher on the telephone, or meet him or her for an informal interview, ask if remuneration is expected. After all, time is a valued commodity.

Interview Questions

There are certain questions you should first ask yourself and other questions more appropriate for you to ask your potential teacher. Also, be prepared to answer any questions from the teachers you might interview. Keep in mind that the interview can go either way. You might decide to back out first if you sense that a good student–teacher relationship might not be possible, or the Reiki teacher might decline to teach you if he or she feels that there is not sufficient rapport between the two of you.

Obviously, the Reiki Master has the final say as to who will or won't become her student. Don't be discouraged if one Reiki teacher refuses you. Consider that it's all for the best, and seek out another possible teacher.

Questions to Ask Yourself

- Does the teacher's gender matter to me? Do I prefer a male or female teacher?
- Am I willing to travel in order to attend a class? If so, how far away from my home am I willing to go?
- How much am I willing to pay for instruction?

Questions to Ask Potential Teachers

- What are your credentials? How long have you been working with Reiki?
- How many attunements do you pass to your students? Do you offer booster attunements?
- Are you available for your students after class? To what extent?
- What materials will I need for your classes?

- What topics do you cover in your classes?
- How much classroom time is instructional, and how much is hands-on practice?
- What are your fees?
- Will I receive a Reiki certificate after completing your class?
- Are you involved in a Reiki group in my area?
- How many students are there in your classes?
- Do you teach all levels of Reiki? What Reiki systems do you teach?

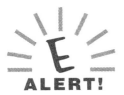

ALERT!

Don't be nervous or dwell for long on any second thoughts about the attunements. You'll get through them all just fine. There is so much more to Reiki than the initial empowerment.

Beyond the Interview

Aside from evaluating the responses each potential teacher gives you in answer to your questions, you should also consider how each individual impressed you overall. With which teacher did you feel most comfortable? Who seemed to be the most knowledgeable? Did any of them seem annoyed by your questions?

First impressions are normally good indicators for how the two of you will get along during the class. After all, how helpful can a person be in answering questions you might have during a class if he or she was brusque or demonstrated irritability while giving responses to your questions during the initial interview?

Preparing for the Attunement

Once you have found your Reiki Master and set up a time for the attunement ceremony, you will need to start preparing your mind and body for the event. Your body should be free of any foods, drinks, and other substances that diminish mental awareness or stimulate the body unnaturally. Drink plenty of water to flush yourself of any lurking toxins. Avoid nicotine, caffeine, recreational drugs, and alcohol for at least twenty-four hours prior to your class. An exception to this rule is to continue taking any prescribed medications according to your health provider's directions.

A full night's sleep prior to your class is recommended, so get to bed early, or at least avoid any late–night activities like watching television into the wee hours of the morning. Be sure to eat a healthy, nutritious breakfast the morning of your class. Fifteen to twenty minutes of meditation in the morning will also help calm you of any nervous jitters or stomach butterflies.

Reiki Initiation Ritual

The Reiki attunement is much anticipated by Reiki students. Attunements have been and still are somewhat cloaked in shadowed secrecy. The Reiki students are requested to keep their eyes shut when the attunements are passed. Naturally, this gives Reiki attunements an air of mystery, implying that the students are not supposed to see what is being done to them. The actual reason that students are asked to keep their eyes closed is to help them achieve a relaxed and meditative state.

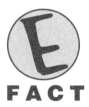

FACT

The attunement process inspires a myriad of feelings and emotions. Every newly attuned practitioner's experience of his or her attunement is unique. It is a personal and intimate experience that some individuals prefer to keep private. Others can barely hold their excitement and will quickly share their Reiki awakening experience with others.

Traditional Usui Reiki Masters give their students four attunements for initiation into Reiki Level I, two attunements for Reiki Level II, and one attunement for Reiki Level III. Attunements for all levels are somewhat similar, but each also has its own slight variation.

In addition to the traditional attunements given by Usui Reiki Masters, there is a powerful and versatile attunement called the Hui Yin. The Reiki Master can use the Hui Yin whenever he or she feels a student is in need of this special attunement. The Hui Yin is also called the booster attunement.

Reiki and Karma

During or after the attunement ceremony, many Reiki practitioners experience the phenomenon of remembering the use of Reiki in a former life. For some, this memory will surface through their conscious wakeful minds, detailing considerable information. Visually sensitive people might actually witness the scenes being played out through images in their mind's eye. At other times the memory enters through the subconscious mind in nighttime dreams.

Some people feel that those who are drawn to Reiki here on earth were predestined to be healers during times when our planet is suffering unrest and afflictions such as war, poverty, and environmental disturbances.

Booster Attunements

Booster attunements are Reiki attunements that can be given to a Reiki practitioner as a turbo-charge to help get Reiki flowing whenever it seems to be dormant or blocked. The Reiki Master can use the Hui Yin attunement as a booster attunement for any level practitioner who has already been attuned to Reiki.

Hui Yin Attunement Preparation

In preparation for passing the Hui Yin attunement to a Reiki practitioner, the Reiki Master kneels down in each corner of the room and cleans the room with the Power symbol by drawing the Cho Ku Rei with sweeping motions in the air using open and flat palms. This can be done prior to the arrival of the attunee.

After the attunee has been seated in the chair, the Reiki Master says a silent prayer to ground and center herself. The Reiki Master acknowledges her own higher self, as well as the higher self of the attunee awaiting the booster attunement. Acknowledgment is also offered to any spirit beings that are recognized as being present. These may include Dr. Usui, Dr. Hayashi, Hawayo Takata, Allah, Buddha, Jesus, Reiki guides, or any other spiritual beings.

The Hui Yin Attunement

The Reiki Master asks the attunee awaiting the booster attunement to close his eyes and to keep them closed until the attunement ritual is completed. Then the Master goes through the following steps to pass the Hui Yin booster attunement.

Step One

The Reiki Master begins by standing in front of the seated attunee. She then walks around the left side of the attunee and stands directly behind the back of the chair, with her feet planted firmly on the floor. The Reiki Master should stand with her feet shoulder-width apart and her knees slightly bent. This stance must be maintained so that the body will not sway.

Step Two

The Reiki Master holds the Hui Yin Position with her tongue pressed against the roof of her mouth. She takes a deep breath and holds it for two to four minutes.

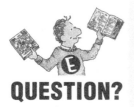

QUESTION?

What is the Hui Yin Position?
In the Hui Yin Position, the Reiki Master contracts muscles of the vagina and anus (or, in the case of male Masters, just the anus), blocking air from entering the vagina and rectum. While holding the Hui Yin, she presses her tongue to the roof of the mouth, with the tip of the tongue slightly touching the gap between the back of the front two teeth. She takes a deep breath and holds it for two to four minutes.

Step Three

This step is done without releasing the Hui Yin Position, as the Reiki Master resumes breathing. In the air over the attunee's crown, she draws the Master symbol, Dai Ko Myo. She silently says "Dai Ko Myo" three times. She then places her left hand on top of her right hand and makes a semiforceful action of pushing the drawn symbol into the attunee's head, without actually touching his head.

The Reiki Master senses the energy moving down the attunee's body and returning up to the crown. She cups her hands together and holds them over the attunee's head. Cupped hands are parted slightly, creating a small opening. The Reiki Master bends over and blows through the opening in the hands into the top of the attunee's head.

The Hui Yin Position is continued while the Reiki Master passes the following symbols:

- The Reiki Master draws the Power symbol, Cho Ku Rei, over the attunee's crown, as she silently says "Cho Ku Rei" three times. The Master then places her left hand on top of her right hand and makes a semiforceful action of pushing the drawn symbol into the attunee's head, without actually touching his head. The Reiki Master senses the energy moving down the attunee's body and returning up to the crown. The symbol is pushed back into the attunee's head for a second time.

- Next, the Reiki Master draws the Connection symbol, Hon Sha Ze Sho Nen, over the attunee's crown as she silently says "Hon Sha Ze Sho Nen" three times. She then places her left hand on top of her right hand and makes a semiforceful action of pushing the drawn symbol into the attunee's head, without actually touching his head. The Reiki Master senses the energy moving down the attunee's body and returning up to the crown. The symbol is pushed back into the attunee's head for a second time.

- The Master draws the Harmony symbol, Sei Hei Ki, over the attunee's crown. She silently says "Sei Hei Ki" three times. Then, she places her left hand on top of her right hand and makes a semiforceful action of pushing the drawn symbol into the attunee's head, without actually touching his head. The Reiki Master senses the energy moving down the attunee's body and returning up to the crown. The symbol is pushed back into the attunee's head for a second time.

Step Four

Continuing to hold the Hui Yin Position, the Reiki Master walks along the attunee's left side and stands in front of him. She then kneels before the attunee and, while continuing to hold the Hui Yin Position, takes the attunee's hands and holds them so that they are unfolded and with palms facing up. The Reiki Master places her right hand on top of the attunee's dominant hand (usually the right hand) and she places her left hand underneath the attunee's dominant hand. The Reiki Master continues to hold the attunee's dominant hand with her left hand while drawing these Reiki symbols on the attunee's palm with her right hand:

- The Connection symbol, Hon Sha Ze Sho Nen, is drawn on the attunee's dominant palm. The Reiki Master silently says "Hon Sha Ze Sho Nen" three times. With three pats of her right hand, the symbol is placed into the attunee's hand
- The Harmony symbol, Sei Hei Ki, is drawn on the attunee's dominant palm. The Reiki Master silently says "Sei Hei Ki" three times. With three pats of her right hand, the symbol is placed into the attunee's hand.
- The Power symbol, Cho Ku Rei, is drawn on the attunee's dominant palm. The Reiki Master silently says "Cho Ku Rei" three times. With three pats of her right hand, the symbol is placed into the attunee's hand.

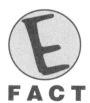

FACT

Reiki symbols are traditionally placed in the dominant hand of the attunee during the Reiki attunement process. If you're right-handed, your right hand is the dominant one. If you're left-handed, it would be your left hand.

If the Hui Yin attunement is given to a Level III practitioner, the Master symbol, Dai Ko Myo, is to be included with the other symbols that are drawn on the attunee's hands in step four.

Step Five

The Reiki Master encloses the attunee's hands with her hands, holding them together in the Gassho Position (the traditional prayer position).

Step Six

The Reiki Master takes a deep breath and blows a stream of breath at the attunee, beginning at the attunee's root chakra and upward to his heart chakra.

Step Seven

The Reiki Master returns to the back of the attunee and closes the attunee's crown aura. This is done with both palms facing down over the head. The palms close the aura by making a circular, counterclockwise motion, similar to the way your hand moves when polishing a table with a cloth.

Step Eight

The Reiki Master releases the Hui Yin Position.

Step Nine

Steps one through eight are repeated for a second time.

Step Ten

The attunement is completed when the Reiki Master draws the Raku symbol in the air directly behind the attunee's back. The Raku is then gently pushed by hand into the attunee's back. The Reiki Master walks to the front of the attunee and places the attunee's hands over his solar plexus and heart. The Reiki Master bows to the attunee in honor of him.

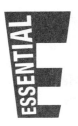

The purpose of using the Reiki Completion symbol, Raku, at the end of the attunement is to close the attunee's auric field that had been opened during the attunement ceremony. The Raku is the serpentine symbol that connects the ground with the sky.

Twenty-One Days of Purification

After receiving a Reiki attunement, an individual will go through the detoxification period. Your body needs to be cleansed both physically and spiritually. Side effects resulting from impurities purged from the physical body are normally more apparent. Diarrhea is commonplace. Also, an unquenchable thirst often occurs to provoke the drinking of large quantities of fluids in order to help flush unhealthy toxins from the body.

While the physical body is going through its purging process, spiritual and mental detoxification is also taking place. The emotional body will release toxins through tears, laughter, coughing, sneezing, and other physically manifested actions. The spiritual body's housecleaning is often expressed by changes in sleep patterns, experiencing vivid dreams, and third-eye openings. The mental body detoxifies when the individual's brain reorganizes his or her thought patterns. It is during this period that self-evaluation takes place.

Coping with Lows and Highs

The lows and highs associated with Reiki's detoxification process can be physically discomforting and emotionally disconcerting. The best way to adjust to any changes that occur is to be as gentle as possible with yourself. Listen to your body and give what it asks for. If you are feeling tired, take a midday nap or go to bed early. If you are craving chocolate, indulge yourself and eat a chocolate bar, or perhaps a small piece of chocolate if you are on a diet. Whatever you do, do not deny your body what it craves.

Do your best to cope with any mood swings that you experience. If you feel like crying, allow the tears to flow naturally without trying to stifle the sobs. If you feel like you need to hug somebody and there is no one around, hug yourself. And don't feel silly. It's really okay to hug yourself. Really!

If you need some alone time and your family is crowding you, pack your bag and check yourself into a hotel room for a couple of days to allow yourself the privacy you need. If the demands of your family don't allow you to escape to a hotel, try some other creative ways to achieve solace, even if only for short periods. Lock yourself inside the bathroom and take a soothing warm soak in the tub. Or you can instruct your family members that whenever you are wearing a particular article of clothing, it signifies that you wish to be left alone. The article you wear should be something that can easily be attached and removed as needed, such as a scarf tied around your neck or a sash around your waist.

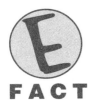

FACT

The detoxification period that follows a Reiki attunement is symbolically called the "Twenty-One-Day Purification Period." However, this period may be shorter or, more rarely, longer than twenty-one days.

Who Wants to Feel Sick?

After reading about the discomforts and mood swings that can occur during the detoxification period that follows an attunement, you might be wondering why anyone would even want to sign up for a Reiki class. Why put yourself through all that pain? Who wants to feel sick? Is there an upside to all this? Do the benefits truly outweigh the possible hardships suffered along the way?

In response to these questions, consider the following. In less than a month's time, your body will become cleared of all those impurities that most likely took you years to accumulate. Having a Reiki attunement is like pushing the speed-dial button on your telephone. It transmits quickly, cutting through any garbling static in the wiring. There is never a wrong number dialed. Reiki knows where to go and how to make the right connection. The connecting party is you.

Each Reaction Is Different

Although the attunement process is the same for everyone, it affects each person in a different way. Some people will glide through the purification period with barely any noticeable changes. Others are not so fortunate and will go through a more difficult adjustment. It all depends on what condition the student is in prior to the attunement. If you tend to bury your emotions, Reiki will push them to the surface in order to force you to deal with them in the open. If you were suffering from a flu infection that had not yet run its course, Reiki would magnify all your symptoms (chills, fever, and headache) and advance their progression through your body more quickly. This means that you will perhaps suffer from these symptoms more intensely, but the flu will burn itself out in one or two days, rather than linger in your body for a longer period of time.

Similar to Reiki attunements, Reiki treatments can also speed up healing in this same manner. This is why some people will report that they felt worse after receiving a Reiki treatment than they did before the treatment. If there are active imbalances in your body that are menacing to your health, those imbalances can become exaggerated when Reiki is given. Symptoms might quickly heighten to greater degrees than they would have otherwise. But, on the positive side, with Reiki's assistance, those imbalances, magnified or not, will pass entirely out of the body much sooner than expected.

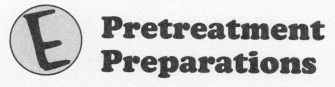

Chapter 5

Pretreatment Preparations

Reiki can be done with no preparation whatsoever when treating emergency conditions or providing quick anxiety relief during times of trauma. However, when applying a full-body Reiki treatment, it is beneficial for the Reiki practitioner to take a few simple steps in preparation. Preparedness helps the Reiki practitioner with focus and intent and helps the recipient to feel more relaxed and be more receptive to healing.

Reiki Principles

The Reiki Principles are the spiritual ideals of the practice of Reiki. Dr. Mikao Usui, the founder of the Usui Reiki System of Healing, added the five principles to the Reiki teachings when he realized that Reiki encompassed much more than just the physical aspects of healing. Dr. Usui was a spiritual man. He valued daily prayer and ethical behavior, and he believed that by living the Reiki Principles, a harmonious life would result.

Repeating the Reiki Principles daily serves as a basic preparation for treating yourself and others as they should be treated. There are many variations of the Reiki Principles in print. Here is one version:

- Just for today, I will not be angry.
- Just for today, I will not worry.
- Just for today, I will give thanks for my many blessings.
- Just for today, I will do my work honestly.
- Just for today, I will be kind to my neighbor and every living thing.

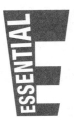

The Reiki Principles are spiritual ideals loosely based on the Buddhist teaching to live in the moment with the understanding that it is not what happens to us in life that upsets us but our reactions to life circumstances that can bring about upsets. Living the principles will help you achieve inner peace and harmony.

Cleansing Your Body Temple

Your body serves as the vessel through which Reiki flows to another person. For this reason it is important that your body is clean, well groomed, and nourished when you're giving a treatment.

Shower or bathe your body, brush your teeth, and assure that your breath is freshened before the arrival of the person you intend to treat with Reiki. Use natural or unscented deodorants. Avoid wearing perfumes or washing beforehand with scented soaps, since some people are sensitive to the chemicals in these products.

Epsom salts, sea salts, and baking soda are all body purifiers that can be used effectively in the bathtub. Soaking in a tub filled with warm water with any of these or a mixture of them for fifteen to twenty minutes will detoxify your body. A detoxification bath will also draw energy from the body and can make you feel drained afterward. Be sure to replenish your energy by drinking eight to twelve ounces of spring water during and/or after the bath.

Take an Aura Bath

Giving yourself an aura bath is great anytime, but is especially helpful between Reiki sessions. Your aura is like a magnet, picking up vibrational energies that are floating around everywhere you go. It is important to cleanse your aura frequently, freeing it from foreign vibrations and negative energies. Here are three ways to cleanse your aura:

1. Cleanse your hands with cool running water. Then, use your fingers to "comb" through the space surrounding your body, from head to toe. After you're done, cleanse your hands again.
2. Using a single feather or feather whisk made from owl or turkey feathers, make sweeping motions through the space surrounding your body.
3. "Smudge" the area surrounding your body with the smoke from an herbal wand made from white sage, lavender, cedar, and/or sweet grass. (Avoid doing this if you suffer from any respiratory problems.)

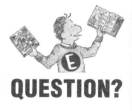

How do I smudge my aura?
Light the smudging wand using a match or candlelight. Blow the flame out or wave the wand to put out the fire. Allow the smudge stick to smolder, freeing the smoke to circle in the air. Holding the herbal wand in one hand, fan the swirls of smoke with your other hand around your body's aura from your head to your toes.

Soak Up Healing Rays

Sit by a sunny window and soak up some healing rays for a few minutes each morning. The sun is a natural healer and will vitalize your body, fend off depression, and keep your energy balanced. If you live in a region where sunshine is sparse, you can substitute light therapy by sitting under special lamps designed for this purpose.

Dress Comfortably

The most appropriate clothing to wear, whether you are the practitioner or the recipient, is anything comfortable and loose fitting. Don't wear nylon pantyhose or any type of clothing that clings to the body too tightly. Garments made from natural fabrics—cottons, silks, and woolens—are more breathable than synthetic materials. Nonporous and clingy synthetic fabrics tend to restrict the flow of Reiki. It is not necessary for recipients to remove apparel for Reiki treatment, but they should take off their shoes and belt.

Reiki recipients should wear cosmetics sparingly or not at all. Also, they should avoid using hairspray. Cosmetics and hairspray can be a hindrance, since the hands of the Reiki practitioner will be touching the recipient's face and head. If the practitioner's hands perspire, it is possible that chemicals from the makeup and hairspray can be transferred to the recipient's clothing when the practitioner uses her hands to apply Reiki to the recipient's torso and back.

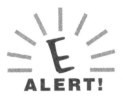

ALERT!

If you are ever asked to remove your clothing to receive a Reiki treatment, immediately consider this an inappropriate request; refuse any further treatment by the practitioner and head straight for the nearest exit. That Reiki practitioner is not to be trusted.

Nourish Your Body

Having optimal health is essential for practicing Reiki, and eating well is essential for optimal health. Eating five or six small-portion meals each day is recommended over eating just two or three large meals. Make healthy food choices and avoid all fast foods, snacks loaded with carbs, and junk foods.

Some healers prefer to fast before treating others because the digestion process can interfere with their personal comfort and overall efficiency when doing healing work. If this is the case, be sure to nourish your body after the Reiki session is over. However, you also don't want to experience hunger during the session. A growling tummy can be a distraction, so a small meal beforehand might be called for. Consuming a piece of fruit, a few celery or carrot sticks, a small handful of almonds, or a small glass of fruit juice or bottled water before a session might be enough to stave off hunger pangs.

Certainly keep any of your meals light prior to giving someone a treatment in order to avoid feeling sluggish or having gastrointestinal discomfort. Avoid eating garlic or anything that can cause offensive breath. Do not drink any alcoholic beverages and avoid all caffeinated drinks for at least twenty-four hours prior to giving Reiki.

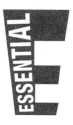

Drink plenty of water. Purified water and natural spring water can hydrate your body and flush out any impurities within it. It is important that both practitioner and recipient drink a full glass of water immediately following a full-body treatment.

A Healing Space

It is meaningful to have a space dedicated to healing. Whether you have a room designated solely for Reiki treatments or only temporarily set up an area as a Reiki space in your home, honor your healing space by keeping it clean and uncluttered. Televisions and telephones have no place in your healing space. Turn the television off and turn off the ringer on your phone.

If you cannot turn off the telephone, inform the Reiki recipient that your answering machine will record any calls if your phone rings and that the Reiki session will not be interrupted. The Reiki session should always be your first priority. Avoid any distractions that might arise suddenly. Taking a phone call or answering the doorbell in the middle of a healing session would give the Reiki recipient the message that he or she is clearly not your first priority.

Reiki Equipment and Supplies

Keep all your equipment and related supplies close at hand. Here is a list of recommended items to have available:

- **Massage table**—You can use a bed, couch, or recliner to give a full-body Reiki treatment, but a massage table is the most comfortable choice. There are many portable tables on the market. The standard width is 29 inches. The standard height is adjustable from 22 to 35 inches. You can expect to pay from $300 to $500, depending on the table model that best fits your needs.
- **Face rest**—The face rest is an accessory to your massage table. It allows the Reiki recipient to lie face down on his stomach. Without the face rest, the recipient will need to have his neck turned to the right or left, which can cause discomfort after a prolonged period of time. You can also purchase washable covers for the face rest, providing additional comfort and hygiene.
- **Chair**—You will need a chair or stool to sit on when giving a Reiki treatment. An armless desk chair with wheels or a swivel stool are both good choices so that you can roll back and forth as needed when positioning your hands.
- **Bolster**—A bolster is used to relieve stress from the lower-back region. Keep it tucked under the Reiki recipient's knees while she is lying on her back. A smaller one can also be tucked under the recipient's ankles when she is lying on her stomach. A makeshift bolster can easily be made by rolling up a large, soft towel.
- **Blanket**—Keep a blanket or two nearby to cover the person you are treating in case he complains of feeling chilled.
- **Pillows**—Most recipients prefer to have a pillow cushioning their head, or perhaps a small rolled-up hand towel under the neck, rather than lying with their head flat on the table surface. Pillows can also be used as arm rests for the practitioner. A firm pillow placed on the practitioner's lap will provide much-needed comfort and prevent

cramping or shaking as the practitioner stretches her arms across the table and over the recipient's body.

- **Other items**—Additional supplies to have readily on hand are clean linens, tissues, a wastebasket, and bottled water.

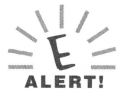

ALERT!

Be sure both the practitioner and the recipient use the bathroom before beginning a Reiki session. A full-body treatment can last from one to two hours, and it is best if neither of you interrupt the session.

With Healing Intentions

Healing can be strengthened when there is a clear goal to reach. Setting an intention before the treatment begins helps to focus the energy used in healing. It is important that the practitioner has a clear understanding of the reasons why the recipient has requested a Reiki healing. That way, both the practitioner and the recipient are focused on the same outcome.

Sometimes it is not clear as to why a treatment is needed. When this is the case, the practitioner could suggest that the first treatment be focused on the recipient receiving clarity as to what his most significant needs are. Using "receiving clarity" as an intention can be very powerful in getting directly to any illness or imbalance within the body.

The Gassho Ritual

Gassho (pronounced "gash sho") is the act of bringing the hands together in a prayerlike fashion in front of the heart. It is used as an acknowledgment, a prayerful greeting of sorts. In using Gassho, the Reiki practitioner is recognizing the source of the healing energies and is thanking the Creator for the opportunity to serve as a vessel for Reiki to flow through. Gassho is often done for a few brief seconds before the session begins and again at the end of the session. The healing intention that was selected for the session can be stated out loud during the Gassho ritual at the start of the Reiki treatment.

Curbing Your Expectations

Setting an intention is very different from having an expectation. An intention is a focus that empowers healing, allowing it to unfold naturally. An expectation tends to limit healing because holding an expectation is a form of rigid control and involves passing judgment.

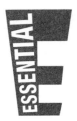

Charge up your battery by nourishing your body and doing whatever needs to be done to offer the best help you can. But, aside from that, there is nothing more you can do. Setting up expectations is really only setting up yourself and the recipient for failure.

Being able to put aside your expectations and accepting whatever happens in a healing session is not always easy. As healers, we want to help heal people's dis-eases, but placing an expectation on the "when" or "how" a person will heal is actually a controlling mechanism. We are not in control of anyone's healing journey. We are only facilitators, willing to act as tools.

When you expect someone to get better and they don't, you will feel bad and blame yourself. If you expect nothing and the recipient doesn't get better, you may still feel bad, but you won't blame yourself for the failure of achieving something you expected.

Centering and Grounding

Each one of us has a unique personality, and so we often get caught up in the illusion that we are totally separate beings. But in reality, each of us is only a miniscule part of the whole. We are a part of the universe, not something outside of the universe. Our egos want to keep us isolated from one another when we place overt importance on our differences. However, we can appreciate and celebrate our individual uniqueness without isolating ourselves from the universe.

It is the power of the universal source that sustains us. Yoga and tai chi are two excellent exercise methods that can help align your energies with the universe. Meditation and visualization are other ways that help to center and ground our energies.

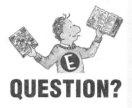

QUESTION?

What is a grounded person?
A person whose energetic soul-body is in synch with the physical body is grounded. If you are emotionally charged, either by expression (anger, frustration, sadness) or by experience (bewilderment, distraction, confusion), you are ungrounded, with your soul drifting away to another place. Being accident-prone is an obvious characteristic of being ungrounded.

Grounding Exercises

There are many guided-meditation CDs and videos on the market that can help you become centered and grounded. Look for taped meditations that are meant for chakra alignment or for grounding yourself. Following are a couple of scripted meditations that you can try.

Earth-Grounding Meditation

You are barefoot, sitting on a stone bench alongside a grassy hillside. Focus on your feet. They are touching the ground beneath you. Imagine roots shooting out from the soles of your feet and your toes. Imagine the roots spreading wider and deeper into the soil. These roots enable you to draw into your body the positive energies of the Mother Earth.

Your feet have now sunk into the moist dirt. Wiggle your toes in your comfortable earthy slippers. Notice your ankles being tickled by the tall grasses blowing in a gentle wind. Feel the blood pumping through the veins in your legs.

Feel your buttocks planted firmly on the cool stone bench. Move your hips slightly from side to side, allowing your body to adjust to the natural curvature of the stone. You are now a part of this stone. You are feeling very relaxed.

Relax your breathing. The deeper you breathe, the more relaxed you feel. Continue to take slow, deep breaths. Deep . . . deep . . . deeper.

Listen to the constant pulse of your heartbeat. Let the sound of the steady beat of your heart drop to your solar plexus. Belly in. Belly out. Belly in. Belly out.

Release any tension in your back. Allow your torso to slump slightly. Every movement you make releases more and more tensions from your body. Move your shoulders slightly forward. Allow your head to wobble gently from side to side. Tip your head to the right. Now tip it to the left. Drop your chin to your chest. Allow your head to bob up and down slowly. Allow your head to wobble naturally, with no jerky motions.

Lift your head. Close your eyes. Focus on your eyelids. Notice the flutter of your lashes against the soft tissues under your eyes. Keeping your eyes shut, allow yourself to notice the movements of your eyeballs. Are they still? Are they moving? Don't force them to do anything—just let them be.

Take your hands and allow your fingers to walk across your scalp and through your hair. Imagine that this tingling sensation is awakening your brain and stimulating your thought processes. Comb your hair with your fingers. Don't worry about messing up your hairstyle. You are now clearing away any debris from your aura that is obstructing your crown chakra. By doing this you are clearing a pathway for you to feed from the universe's unlimited healing energies. With your feet planted deeply into the earth and your crown open to the white light pouring down through your crown chakra into your whole being, you are now aligned with the Creator and ready to begin.

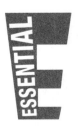

You can record your own meditation tapes, which you can play back for yourself to guide you through the meditation. Here are a few tips you may find useful: Pretest the recorder's volume setting before recording. As you record your voice, speak slowly and enunciate. Use a high-quality tape to reduce sound distortion.

Ocean-Grounding Visualization

Imagine that you are lying inside a glass-bottomed boat that is floating over the deep blue ocean waters. You are lying on your belly, looking down toward the ocean floor. There are many colorful fish swimming in the water beneath you. You are safe in the boat, yet you feel as if you are very much a part of the marine life—the coral reefs, seaweed, fish, and sea turtles. You can feel the boat rocking gently to the rhythmic motion of the ocean waves.

A school of dolphins now appears. As they are swimming along playfully, they begin to breach the water near the boat, splashing salty water onto the deck. You are now wet and laughing. You slip out of the boat and are now swimming among the carefree dolphins.

Any worries or concerns you have are fading away quickly as you immerse yourself totally into the fluidity of the ocean. You are filled with joy and peace, reveling in the moment. You are now floating on top of the water, looking up at the sky and basking in the feel of the sun on your skin. Perfection.

Soon the dolphins swim away, into deeper waters. You are now swimming toward the shore. Within a few arm strokes, your feet touch the sand on the bottom. You stand upright and walk up onto the sandy beach.

You are now sitting in the wet sand near the water's edge. You are building a magnificent sandcastle. The tide begins to roll in and your beautiful sandcastle is being washed away. You are now lying upon the sand, allowing the tidal waters to flood over your body with its continuing waves.

As you are lying on the sand with the water rushing over you, you realize that you are a part of the sand. You realize you are a part of the water. You also realize you are a part of the air above you. You are aware that you are a part of everything and that you are no longer feeling as if you are a separate being. Not ever a separate being, you now know that you are always part of the whole.

Are You Ready?

In order for a Reiki treatment to be most effective, it is absolutely essential that the practitioner make all necessary preparations beforehand. A calm, clean, and uncluttered environment for the treatment is essential.

Physical needs, such as basic hygiene and nourishment requirements, must be given close attention. To make sure both the practitioner and the recipient are grounded and centered, you may meditate prior to starting a session. Lastly, an intention statement, or prayer request, should be made to indicate the purpose of the session. And after that, it's time to move on to the Reiki hand placements. Ⓔ

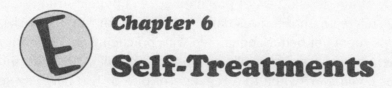

Chapter 6
Self-Treatments

Practicing Reiki through self-treatments helps to process and sustain the positive changes that an attunement to Reiki promises. When you are ill, self-treatments will help bring you back to good health. When you are healthy, self-treatments will reinforce your vitality and strengthen your immune system. Giving a Reiki self-treatment is easy—all you need are your hands, your body, and a willingness to heal and be healed.

A Regular Reiki Routine

Welcome Reiki into your life by making self-treatments a regular routine. Regularly practicing Reiki enhances other daily routines health-minded individuals incorporate into their lives—personal grooming, eating a healthy diet, practicing meditation, and exercising at the gym.

Newly attuned Reiki Level I practitioners will benefit from doing full-body self-treatment sessions daily for the first four to six weeks. This helps them get better acquainted with practicing Reiki, and it also helps them become energetically and physically balanced. After those first weeks, you can switch to a regimen of one or two full-body self-treatments each week. How often you do Reiki self-treatments is entirely up to you. More is better than less, and less is better than none at all.

A Time Commitment

Please make time to carry out full treatments—you are worth it! Experiment by giving yourself treatments at different times to determine what hours of the day best suit your personal routine.

Early risers who do Reiki in the mornings have discovered that starting off their day with a treatment helps their day run more smoothly and harmoniously. Reiki helps them feel better equipped to confront their problems and deal with those life hurdles that get in their way from time to time.

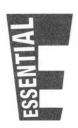

Our lifestyles do not always allow us the luxury of doing Reiki in a quiet or relaxing setting. Rather than forego Reiki altogether, it is better to do Reiki wherever you can, regardless of the environment. Reiki will work on the bus or the subway, and even in the middle of rush hour, if that's where you happen to be at the time it is called for.

Night owls, on the other hand, may mind getting up an hour earlier to perform a treatment. It could make them cranky and more tired.

If your body craves sleep, it will not be open to the idea of being awakened to apply Reiki. It seems self-defeating to forcibly awaken a slumbering body for the sake of applying a relaxation technique. Midmornings and afternoons are often the best times for Reiki if your workday allows either or both.

Doing self-treatments at bedtime can be a good option if you are experiencing insomnia or are sleep-deprived, since Reiki can help lull you to sleep. However, a time when your body is already relaxing is probably not the most favorable time for a Reiki session, because Reiki's relaxing properties can put you to sleep before you've finished the treatment.

Think about your daily schedule and how you function best. Once you've established the time of day most conducive to your lifestyle, commit to doing your self-treatments until it becomes a regular habit.

Relaxing with Reiki

Preferably, Reiki treatments are done in solitude, either in quietness or with soft music being played in the background. Including Reiki self-treatments in an already hectic and time-squeezed schedule doesn't mean you have to sacrifice other activities that you enjoy. Your Reiki self-treatments can be incorporated into other relaxing practices that are already a part of your routine. Here are some ideas:

- Perform Reiki self-treatments while you are reclining on the couch watching television or listening to music.
- Integrate your meditation time with your Reiki treatment.
- Give yourself Reiki while soaking in a hot bubble bath.

Preparing for a Full-Body Session

You don't need much to perform a full-body Reiki session on yourself. During the treatment, you can lie down on a bed, couch, reclining chair, or a clean, carpeted floor. It is absolutely essential that you make certain that you are as comfortable as possible before and during treatment. A full-body Reiki treatment will take roughly sixty to ninety minutes to complete.

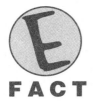

FACT

The mineral zeolite offers an excellent complementary energy for Reiki. According to *Love Is in the Earth: A Kaleidoscope of Crystals* by Melody, its purpose is to promote one's actions and to stimulate the appropriate response to the energies when applied.

Room Temperatures

Make certain that the room you choose for your Reiki sessions is temperature-controlled. It should be heated or cooled to match your personal comfort level. Keep a light wrap or blanket nearby with which to cover yourself in case you feel chilled at any time during the treatment. Reiki energies tend to produce heat, but influxes of both hot and cold temperatures can occur throughout the session. As the Reiki session progresses, you may be surprised to experience a change from the coolness of an air-conditioned room to an atmosphere of coziness and warmth.

Your Reiki Hands

Wash your hands thoroughly before you begin. You may want to remove any rings or bracelets from your fingers and wrists, especially if you are sensitive to the vibrational energies of gold, silver, or gemstones. When you place your hands on your body, be gentle, gentle, gentle! No pressure needs to be applied, since it is the exchange of ki energies that effectively does the healing work for you. When you place your hands, palms facing downward, onto your body, Reiki will begin to flow automatically. It is as simple as that.

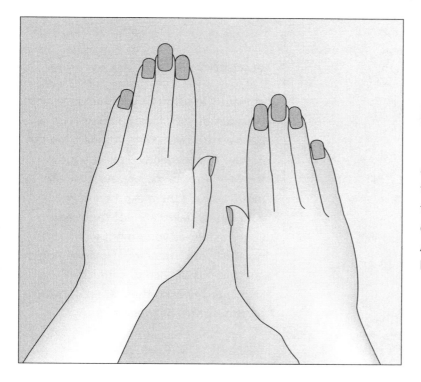

REIKI HANDS

◀ When you use your hands to administer Reiki, hold the fingers and thumbs of each of your hands snugly together so there are no obvious gaps or spaces between them. Remember: All you need is a light touch to get the ki flowing.

Basic Hand Placements

The newly attuned Reiki Level I practitioner should carry out a precise sequence of hand placements during each full treatment. Always begin at the face placement and move downward. Devote five minutes to each placement in order to make sure you don't neglect any part of your body and so that each body part is given equal consideration. Wear a watch or place a clock within your visual range so that you can closely monitor the time spent on each placement.

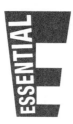

After practicing the hand placements in the traditional sequences for a period of time, it's possible that you will deviate from them to some degree and begin to acquire your own methodology in placing your hands on your body while listening to your inner dialogue.

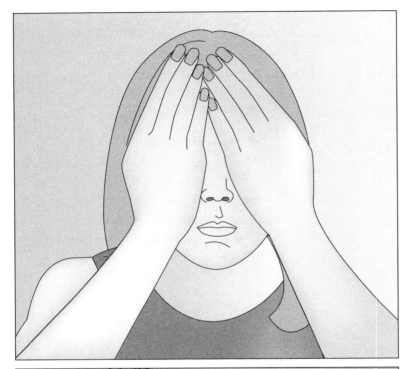

PLACEMENT 1: FACE

◀ Place the palms of your hands against the sides of your face, cupping your hands softly over your eyes. Rest the tips of your fingers gently against your forehead. Do not cover your nose and mouth—leave them exposed between your hands. Take care not to squeeze your nostrils, as you do not want to obstruct your breathing. Hold the fingers and thumbs of each of your hands snugly together so there are no obvious gaps or spaces between them.

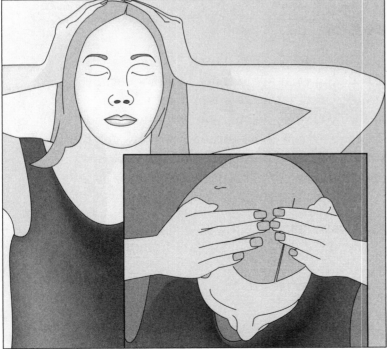

PLACEMENT 2: CROWN AND TOP OF THE HEAD

◀ Take your hands and place the base of each palm just slightly above your ears. Wrap both your palms and fingers along your skull, so that your fingertips meet at the crown.

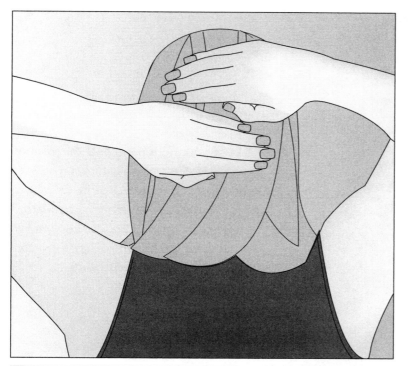

PLACEMENT 3: BACK OF THE HEAD

◀ Cross your arms behind your head, placing one hand on the back of your head and the other directly below it and just above the nape of your neck.

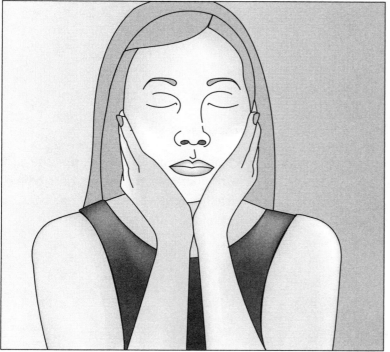

PLACEMENT 4: CHIN AND JAW LINE

◀ Cup your chin and jaw line in your hands, so that your inner wrists touch beneath your chin. Gently rest your fingertips over your earlobes.

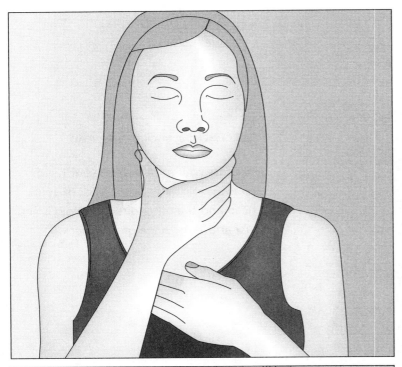

PLACEMENT 5: NECK, COLLARBONE, AND HEART

◄ Place your right hand over the front of your neck, grasping your throat gently while allowing your neck to be held inside the space between your outward-extended thumb and fingers. Rest your left hand on top of your chest, between your collarbone and your heart.

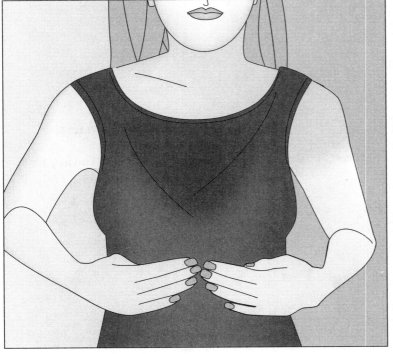

PLACEMENT 6: RIBS

◄ Place your hands on your rib cage, just below your breasts, with your fingertips touching. Your elbows should be bent back a little.

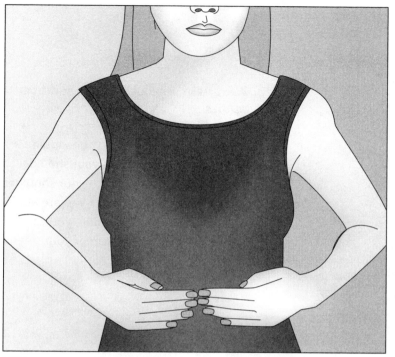

PLACEMENT 7: ABDOMEN

◀ Place your hands on your solar plexus area, just above your navel. Keep your elbows bent and allow your fingertips to touch.

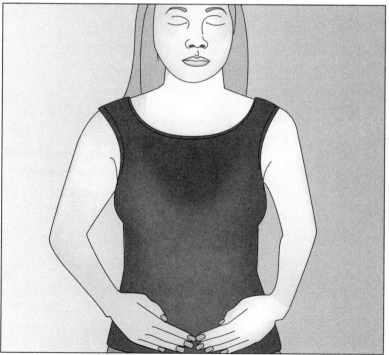

PLACEMENT 8: PELVIC BONES

◀ Place your right hand over your right pelvic bone and place your left hand over your left pelvic bone, so that your fingertips touch in the center.

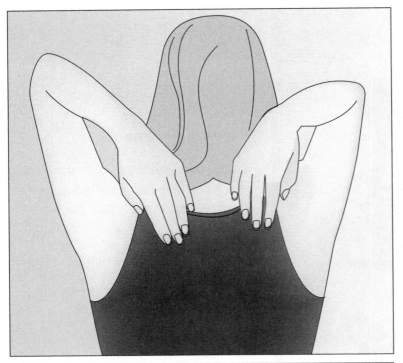

PLACEMENT 9: SHOULDERS AND SHOULDER BLADES

◄ Reach over the top of your shoulders and place your hands on your shoulder blades. If you cannot reach your shoulder blades, reach only as far as you are able to comfortably. As an option, you can rest your hands on the top of your shoulders.

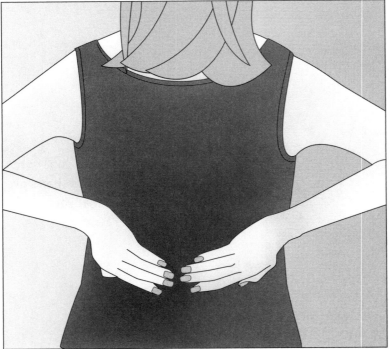

PLACEMENT 10: MIDBACK

◄ Reach behind your back, elbows bent, and place your hands on the middle of your back. Allow your fingertips to touch, if you are able to do so comfortably.

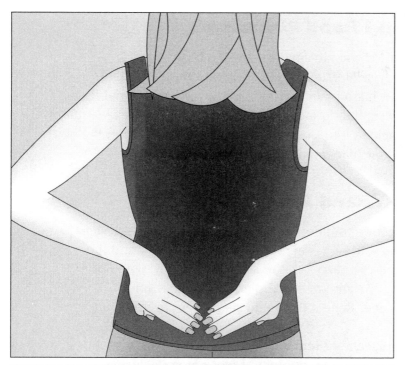

PLACEMENT 11: LOWER BACK

◀ Reach behind your back, elbows bent, and place your hands on your lower back. Allow your fingertips to touch, if you are able to do so comfortably.

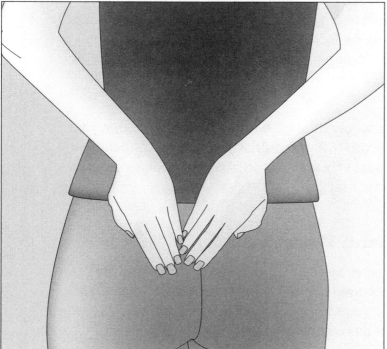

PLACEMENT 12: SACRUM

◀ Reach behind your back, elbows bent, and place your hands on your sacral region.

Traditional Usui Reiki Hand Placements

The Usui System of Natural Healing uses twelve basic hand placements in a full-body self-treatment. (In addition, there are other variations and alternative hand placements offered by nontraditional Reiki systems.) The twelve basic hand placements that are used in giving a full-body Reiki treatment include four placements on the head, four on the front of the body, and four placements on the back of the body.

Nontraditional Reiki Hand Placements

In addition to the twelve traditional Reiki hand placements for self-treatment, you may also add two others—the knee placement and the ankle-and-foot placement. To carry out the knee placement, place one hand over the top of your right knee and place your other hand underneath the same knee. Repeat this hand placement to treat your left knee.

The ankle-and-foot placement requires that you bend your knee in order for your hands to reach your ankle and foot comfortably. Place your left palm on the inside of your left foot, over the anklebone, fingers curled around the top of the foot. At the same time, grasp the sole of your right foot with your right hand. Reverse these hand placements to treat your left foot and right ankle.

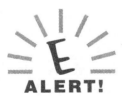
ALERT!

Take your time and follow through with each placement that you are able to make. If you rush too quickly through Reiki's hand placements, you could very well be forfeiting the healing benefits of the hand placement set.

Is It Okay to Skip Hand Placements?

Some people may complain that a particular placement is difficult to carry out or maintain for five minutes—for instance, the shoulder blades and back placements. If you cannot reach these areas, it is okay for you to skip them. The hand placements are taught as guidelines and are not set in stone. Reiki Level II practitioners can send distant Reiki to their own body parts that are unreachable. For more information on sending distant Reiki, see Chapter 8.

Is It Working?

Each person will experience a Reiki session differently. Some people don't feel much of anything. If that's the case with you, keep in mind that just because you don't feel anything, it doesn't mean that nothing is happening. Trust that Reiki is working and continue to move through the different hand placements.

Other people will notice shifts of energies occurring. You may notice your palms are generating pulsing energies, or you may sense energy fluctuations pulsing through your entire body as it receives the ki vibrations.

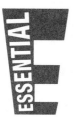

It is normal for Reiki to flow better in some placements than others, or, at times, to not flow at all. Anytime you feel as if the flow of Reiki is blocked, taking a few deep breaths can help start it flowing again.

Like Water from a Spigot

Visualize water flowing from a spigot at different velocities into a basin below it. The flow of the water is determined according to the adjustment of the spigot's knob. When the knob is shut tightly, it blocks water from running out. However, when the knob is turned in varying increments, it allows the water to drip, trickle in a thin stream, or gush out quickly.

Reiki flows from the palms into your body similar to the way water runs from a spigot into a basin, but with Reiki the flow is not dependent on the spigot's knob adjustment. Reiki flows, or doesn't flow, according to the level of acceptance or needs of the basin. In doing self-treatments, your body is the basin that needs filling, and the palms of your hands, facilitating the healing energies, represent the spigot.

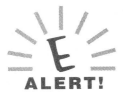
ALERT!

There is nothing sexual about touching yourself when applying Reiki. In applying self-treatments it is perfectly acceptable to touch your breasts and genitalia. But it is not acceptable to touch someone else's private parts when you are treating them.

Reiki on the Fly

It is not always feasible to do a full self-treatment when time constraints and unplanned events interfere. Sometimes, doing a brief spot treatment is more convenient. More is better than less, but less is better than none at all, as long as you avoid making a habit of choosing spot treatments in place of a full-body treatment for the sake of convenience.

A partial treatment can be done while you are sitting upright. Anytime you are sitting and your hands are free, you can quickly apply partial treatments. Do Reiki on yourself when you are:

- Riding on the bus, train, or airplane
- Riding in a car, as long as you're not driving
- Sitting in the dental chair
- Sitting in the theater
- Sitting in a waiting room
- Watching television

Interval Treatments

Another way of dealing with a busy schedule is to make sure you do each of the twelve hand placements for at least five minutes at different intervals throughout the day. Map out your daily activities and combine them in partnership with the different hand placements so that they are done simultaneously each day. Here is a sample schedule of interval treatments for all twelve hand placements:

- **Placement 1, face:** Shortly after waking up in the morning and before getting out of bed

- **Placement 2, crown and top of the head:** In the morning, when you take a shower (You can do this placement as you stand in the hot streaming water.)
- **Placement 3, back of the head:** While sitting at the breakfast table before or after you have your first meal of the day
- **Placement 4, chin and jaw line:** When you get into your car to drive to work or for errands, either before you start the engine or while the engine is warming up (After the session, you'll be able to drive to your workplace in a state of peace and tranquility.)
- **Placement 5, neck, collarbone, and heart:** At lunchtime (If you are eating at a restaurant, you can do it after you've ordered and are waiting for your lunch to be served.)
- **Placement 6, ribs:** Midafternoon, while you are sitting at your desk or at the coffee break table
- **Placement 7, abdomen:** While sitting in the car before you drive home from your workplace
- **Placement 8, pelvic bones:** While you are sitting during your ten-minute meditation practice
- **Placement 9, shoulders and shoulder blades:** While sitting at the kitchen table prior to preparing your evening meal
- **Placements 10, 11, and 12, midback, lower back, and sacrum:** In the evening, either while you are reclining and watching television or while relaxing in your bed before going to sleep

Tracking Your Progress

Keeping inventory of your sessions is an excellent way to track your successes and "failures" (there really are no actual "failures" in healing—noncures are opportunities for us to look at our dis-eases from a different perspective). A chart or graph works really well in keeping your notes orderly.

More journal ideas and other record-keeping information for your personal Reiki experiences can be found in Chapter 14.

On the following page, you can find a sample Self-Treatment Chart.

A Sample Self-Treatment Chart				
Date	**Type of Treatment**	**Pain/Issue**	**Other Treatments**	**Results**
April 15	full treatment	anxiety; heart palpitations	prescribed beta-blocker	calmness; lowering of energies; balanced breath
April 23	spot treatment	toothache	none	numbing relief
April 27	full treatment	routine	none	relaxed mood
May 1	full treatment	indigestion; nausea	ginger tea	neutralized gastric upset
May 6	full treatment	routine	none	fell asleep midsession
May 15	spot treatment	onset of migraine	none	minimal relief

Are You Avoiding Self-Treatments?

If you find yourself avoiding Reiki self-treatments, ask yourself why. People sometimes make excuses for not doing self-treatments because they, consciously or unconsciously, feel unworthy of love and healing. Perhaps they originally signed up to take a class and were attuned to Reiki because they wanted to have a means to extend love and healing to others. What these individuals have yet to fully comprehend is that in avoiding self-treatments, they are hindering their potential to help others.

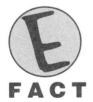
FACT

Reiki's ki energy carries many different names: God Power, Universal Life Energy, Breath of the Great Spirit, Divinity, and Cosmic Energy, among others. There is an unlimited supply of Reiki available for us to tap into.

Although Reiki practitioners are often referred to as healers, they are merely facilitators of healing energies. This means that you, in your role as a Reiki practitioner, have no power to heal others. Rather, you serve a supportive role, assisting another person in his or her healing journey.

Ask yourself why you are willing to assist others in their journeys to heal but are reluctant to support your own journey toward wellness.

Reiki Is a Two-Way Street

Anytime you give a Reiki treatment to someone else, in essence you also receive a healing yourself. That is how Reiki works, plain and simple, because the Universal Life Force first has to be made available through you before the recipient, upon whom you lay your hands, can accept it. Reiki will inherently break through any obstructions in your body that are possibly hampering effective delivery of balancing ki energies to the other person.

You may ask, "If giving Reiki to others helps them and also helps clear away blockages or congestion within my own body, why not skip self-treatments altogether?" Never doing self-treatments and relying solely on treating others as a means to clear your own issues is not the most efficient or loving course of action to take when serving others. Purposely choosing not to do Reiki self-treatments and to give Reiki only to others is denying yourself deeper levels of active healing. The Reiki that flows through you while you are giving someone else a treatment is outwardly focused—after all, the intent is for Reiki to flow through you. Reiki will clear any blockages in your body that are obstructing the pathway to get to the other person, but it will not disperse into the deeper places that need healing within you.

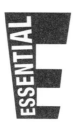

Routinely doing self-treatments is fundamental to Reiki. A practitioner will become more and more comfortable with his or her whole being each time the Reiki hand placements are applied during full-body self-treatments.

In treating others, Reiki's role is a passive one, whereas in applying self-treatments, Reiki takes on a more active role. Routinely doing self-treatments will help keep your ki passageways free of any toxins that accumulate in your body from day to day and will also allow Reiki to penetrate more deeply into your body to negate any imbalances. Regular self-treatment practices will also allow you to assist others in a more loving and balanced manner when you, in turn, give Reiki to them.

Swapping Reiki Treatments

Another way to become more comfortable in doing self-treatments is to meet with another practitioner once a week and swap treatments. At each meeting, two full-body sessions will be completed. You will give one treatment and, in return, be given one treatment. Teaming with another practitioner to swap treatments is a fair exchange that will help open up your body to self-treatments. You can learn more information about exchanging Reiki energies with other practitioners in Chapter 9. Ⓔ

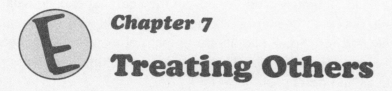

Chapter 7

Treating Others

Open communication between the Reiki practitioner and the recipient is extremely important. When the practitioner and recipient agree to team up as giver and receiver of healing, the two individuals form a special bond, a sort of contractual relationship. While the individual roles of practitioner and recipient may be played out very differently, the primary goal—to promote relaxation and well-being—remains essentially the same.

Newly Attuned Exuberance

A newly attuned Reiki practitioner will often be very anxious to jump in and get busy giving Reiki to everyone. However, your exuberance may be met with varying degrees of apprehension from friends and family members. Try not to be overzealous in selling the benefits of Reiki. Offer to give Reiki treatments to your friends so they can experience Reiki for themselves, but don't be surprised if your offers meet with suspicion and are politely rejected. Some people are simply not as open to Reiki as others. It may take a while for them to warm up to the idea. Respect their feelings and don't push.

No Guinea Pigs

Once you've identified and confirmed a few people among your circle of family and friends who are willing to allow you to give them a full-body Reiki treatment, be careful not to give them the impression that they're serving as guinea pigs in your Reiki experiments. You also shouldn't imply in any way that you are unsure of your effectiveness in applying Reiki. Certainly, you are new at this, but Reiki will flow proficiently, regardless of those through whom it will flow. Is the measure of a gallon of water any less when it is poured out of a brand-new plastic jug than when it is poured from an aged clay pitcher? Of course not. The same is true of the flow of Reiki. Reiki will flow at the appropriate levels as needed by the Reiki recipient, whether or not the practitioner is a beginner or a more advanced channeler of Reiki.

Practicing Reiki in Varying Capacities

Naturally, your awareness of how Reiki works and your confidence in using Reiki will improve over time. Moreover, as you give more treatments you will come to decide in what way being a Reiki practitioner best serves you. Some Reiki practitioners are content in doing only self-treatments while others are also interested in sharing Reiki among immediate family members and their closest friends and relatives. Still other practitioners are drawn to becoming full-time healers and making their healing practice an integral part of their livelihood.

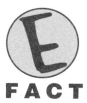

FACT

Oftentimes healers become attuned to Reiki in order to be able to use it as a complementary tool in their occupations as nurses, doctors, chiropractors, herbalists, massage therapists, energy workers, and so on. For some practitioners, Reiki is the precursor that leads to pursuing other health-related occupations.

Pretreatment Communication

It is the responsibility of the Reiki practitioner to help the recipient feel comfortable and reassured before the treatments begin. Be friendly and welcoming. Do your best to address any feelings of anxiety, confusion, or uncertainty that are expressed, either verbally or through body language, and attempt to answer fully all questions that might arise.

It is normal for a person who meets with a Reiki practitioner for the first time to feel a variety of emotions. Among these emotions are excitement, apprehension, expectation, and nervousness. Having someone touch your body, even in a healing atmosphere, can feel like an intrusion of your personal space. Because of this, it is important that the practitioner take some time to help the recipient feel more at ease and establish a level of trust.

Go Over the Treatment Step by Step

Carefully explain the treatment process, delineating exactly what will take place. Naturally, you will not know what your recipient's specific experience may be, as everyone greets Reiki differently. However, you can give an outline of the basic steps that will take place. Here is a list of points you can share with the Reiki recipient before the session begins:

- Approximately how long the treatment will take (sixty to ninety minutes)
- What the recipient needs to do during the treatment (lie on her back for the first part of the treatment and on her stomach for the second part of the treatment)

- How the Reiki recipient will need to be dressed (fully clothed, except for his shoes and belt; loose-fitting attire is preferable)
- Whether it's okay for the recipient to talk, be silent, or even fall asleep during the treatment (It is.)
- How you will touch the recipient's body with your hands during the session (Describe the hand placements and explain that you will begin with the face and move downward.)
- How to breathe during the treatment (Explain that you may ask her to take some breaths from time to time to help the Reiki flow more evenly or to help release blockages.)
- What happens at the end of the treatment (You will comb through the recipient's aura to clear it of stagnant energies that were released from his body.)
- What to do in the next twenty-four hours (The recipient will need to drink plenty of water in order to flush out any toxins that are ready to be eliminated.)

After explaining the treatment step by step, be prepared to answer any additional questions the recipient might have about Reiki and your methodology.

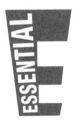

Assure the recipient that Reiki is utterly nonsexual and does not involve any kind of inappropriate touching. If the recipient feels uncomfortable or has any questions at any time during the treatment, be sure he or she understands that it's okay to speak out.

Setting Intentions

As discussed briefly in Chapter 5, pretreatment communication between practitioner and recipient is essential in creating a nurturing atmosphere for healing to occur during a Reiki treatment. Furthermore, it is paramount to a successful Reiki experience that both recipient and practitioner are "on the same page" in regard to what will become the focus of the treatment.

Our life goals are reached most efficiently when the outcomes being sought are clearest in our minds, so communication is key—it is essential to the assurance that both the recipient and practitioner are focused on the same purpose. It would be ideal if, before even arriving for a Reiki treatment, the recipient already had a clear and well-focused intent as to why he or she is seeking the Reiki treatment. But beyond wanting to feel better, most people usually don't have a clear focus as to why they are seeking treatment. Here are a few questions you could ask the recipient to help you both discover a suitable healing intention to use for the treatment:

- How are you feeling today?
- What are your physical health concerns?
- Are you happy?
- Is anything disturbing you?
- What are your expectations for this treatment?
- Do you want to make changes in your perceptions?
- What pushes your emotional buttons?
- What are your current and most troublesome fears?
- Do you have normal sleep patterns?
- Are you an excessive worrier?

These and other similar questions can help pinpoint a specific focus for the Reiki treatment. Prompting the recipient to state his or her intention out loud prior to the treatment can be very effective in helping the focus and flow of Reiki.

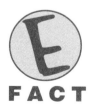

FACT

Reiki practitioners have no legal right to diagnose conditions and should not refer to the people they are treating as patients. However, it is acceptable to urge clients to seek medical advice from a licensed physician regarding symptoms or conditions that are intuited by the Reiki practitioner during treatment.

Hand Placements for Treating Others

The hand placements for giving a Reiki treatment are much like those used for self-treatment. In treating another person, begin at the face placement, complete the other head placements, and move down the body. Allow approximately three to five minutes per hand placement. A full-body treatment normally lasts from sixty to ninety minutes. Again, the hand placements are only guidelines. As you become more proficient, you will learn to place and move your hands intuitively.

It is vital that both the practitioner and the person receiving the treatment are comfortable throughout the session. Make sure you have a comfortable chair or stool, and have the recipient lie on her back upon a massage table. Practitioners will often place one or two pillows upon their laps to help support extended arms as the hand placements are being applied upon the recipient's body. If you do not use a pillow as a prop, your arms and shoulders can become susceptible to discomfort and muscular strain or fatigue, ultimately making your whole body feel tense and sore. Keep your legs apart and your feet planted firmly on the floor. This will help you stay connected to grounding earth energies and keep the flow of Reiki steady.

The First Four Hand Placements

Begin the Reiki treatment with the person lying on his back. Perform Gassho and state the healing intention that was decided on during pretreatment communication. Sit down in a chair directly behind the recipient's head.

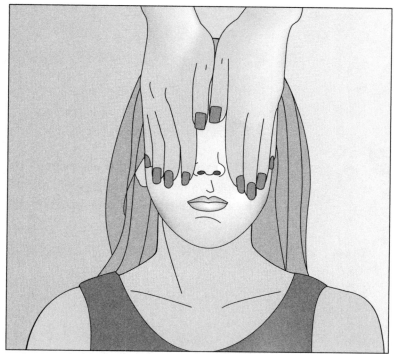

PLACEMENT 1: FACE

◄ Position your hands over the sides of the recipient's face, cupping your fingers lightly over the eyes and placing the palms of your hands gently upon the recipient's forehead. Do not cover the recipient's nose and mouth. Be careful not to squeeze the nostrils—you do not want to obstruct the recipient's breathing.

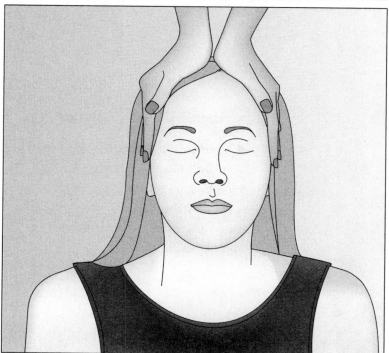

PLACEMENT 2: CROWN AND TOP OF THE HEAD

◄ Place the base of your palms, inner wrists touching, on top of the recipient's head at the crown. Wrap your palms and fingers around the recipient's skull, allowing your fingertips to touch the tops of her ears.

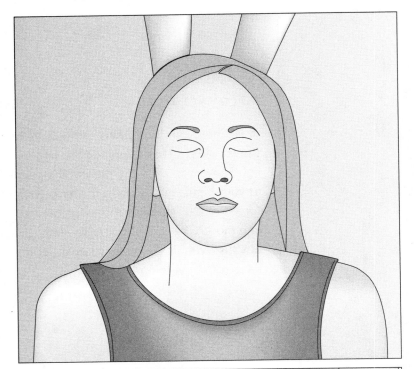

PLACEMENT 3: BACK OF THE HEAD

◄ Slip your hands gently underneath the recipient's head, forming a cradle for the head. Rest the back of your hands on the massage table.

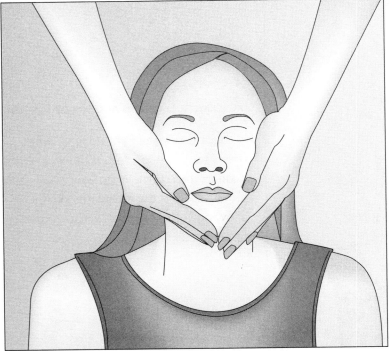

PLACEMENT 4: CHIN AND JAW LINE

◄ Mold your hands gently around the recipient's jaw line, so that your fingertips are touching under the recipient's chin and the heels of your hands are resting beneath her ears or over her earlobes.

Switch Positions for the Next Placement

Placement 5 can be done either while sitting directly behind the recipient's head or sitting at the recipient's side. Choosing where to sit while applying this placement depends on the length of your arms. If your arms are not long enough to comfortably reach the recipient's throat and heart while sitting behind the recipient's head, try moving your chair closer to the side of the table.

PLACEMENT 5: NECK, COLLARBONE, AND HEART

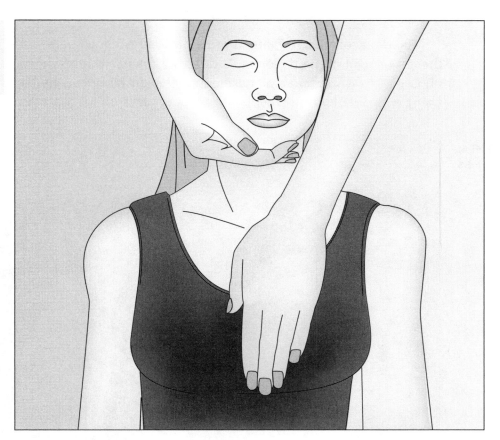

▲ Wrap your right hand around the recipient's neck, allowing the right side of the neck to be held inside the space between your outward-extended thumb and fingers. Alternatively, allow your right hand to hover over the neck. This option is used when the person you are treating feels uneasy about your hand actually touching her throat. Stretch your left arm out and place your left hand over the recipient's heart.

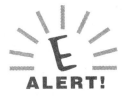

ALERT!

Be especially cautious not to aggravate the recipient by doing a hand placement that might cause sudden pain, stress, or any degree of discomfort. The throat is a sensitive area that many people do not like to have touched because of fears of strangulation or suffocation. Always be sensitive to thoughts and feelings the Reiki recipient might harbor.

The Next Three Hand Placements

Hand placements 6, 7, and 8 are employed while you are sitting to the left or right of the recipient (it does not matter which side you choose). Move your chair alongside the recipient's body as needed. Using a swivel chair on wheels works especially well for this purpose.

PLACEMENT 6:
RIBS

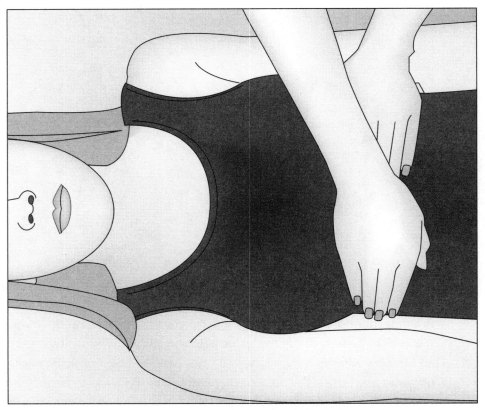

▲ Place your hands on the recipient's rib cage, just below the recipient's breasts.

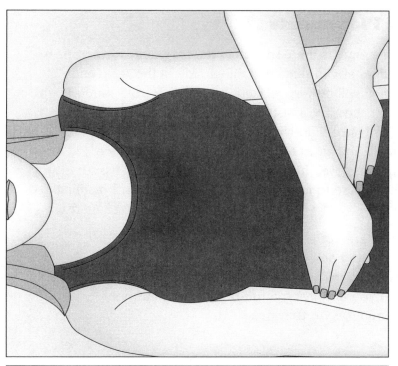

PLACEMENT 7: ABDOMEN

◀ Place your hands on the solar plexus area, above the recipient's navel.

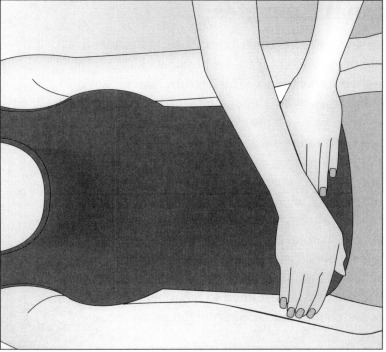

PLACEMENT 8: PELVIC BONES

◀ Place one hand over each of the recipient's pelvic bones.

The Last Four Hand Placements

These final hand placements are done while the recipient is lying on his stomach. The practitioner can remain at either side of the recipient.

It is likely the recipient will be very relaxed, even sleepy, from the Reiki being applied thus far. If necessary, assist the recipient in making the adjustment from lying on his back to lying on his stomach. Attach the face rest to your massage table and assist the recipient in placing his face down. Use a soft cloth-fitted cover, handkerchiefs, or a few facial tissues to cover the face rest, but be sure to leave the center hole open for breathing.

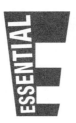

The shoulders are an area of a person's body where you will often sense concentrated amounts of pent-up energy. This is because emotional burdens and worrisome feelings are often stored there. When you are giving a full-body Reiki treatment, spend a few extra minutes on this area.

Blending of Personal Energies

Anytime we are within a few feet of another person, our auras blend together and a fusion of energy takes place. The physical closeness of people can often cause their auras to mix. This, in turn, can create a mixed bag of emotions and sensations. Depending on the circumstances and the relationships between you and the other person, the feelings that surface from energy fusion can range anywhere from pleasingly desirable to fearfully intrusive.

In intimate love relationships, couples welcome the intertwining of their auras, reveling in the energy interchange. Sharing a small office with a coworker is also a situation where auras will blend because of the limited space you share. This can be comfortable or uncomfortable, depending on the two personalities and the extent to which their personalities blend together. In both of these scenarios, because you are familiar with the other person and accustomed to blending your energies, you will adjust and become comfortable in sharing the same space.

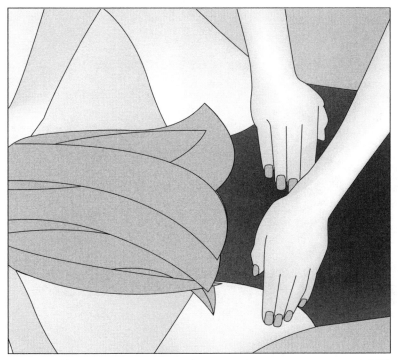

PLACEMENT 9: SHOULDER BLADES

◀ Place your hands on the recipient's shoulder blades.

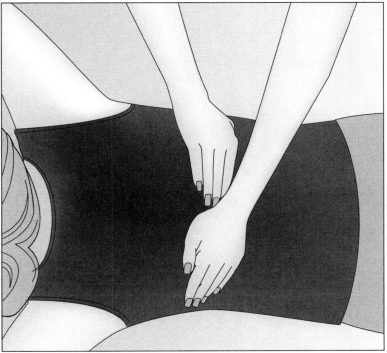

PLACEMENT 10: MIDBACK

◀ Place your hands on the middle of the recipient's back.

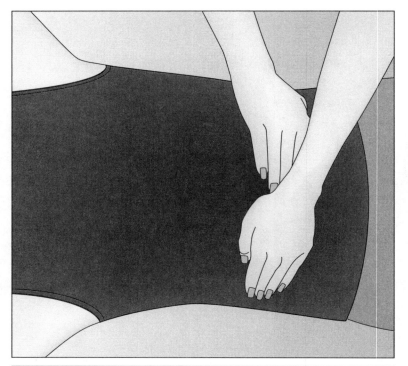

PLACEMENT 11: LOWER BACK

◀ Place your hands on the recipient's lower back.

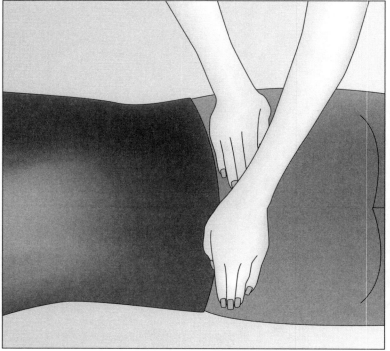

PLACEMENT 12: SACRUM

◀ Place your hands on the recipient's sacral region.

It is often difficult for most of us to share close quarters with total strangers. Consider how you feel when you are in close proximity to a stranger when riding in an elevator or sitting next to a stranger at the movie theater. Most people's auras will shrink closer to their physical bodies as they try to maintain energetic boundaries. During a Reiki session, the auras of the practitioner and recipient will naturally blend. The practitioner not only sits near the recipient, but she actually reaches out and touches the recipient's body.

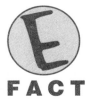

FACT

At the end of the session, the Reiki practitioner combs the recipient's aura to clear it of any energetic debris that has lifted from the physical body during the treatment by moving the hands in multiple circular motions or using feathering sweeps of the hands over the body. As the aura is cleansed, a request is silently made for the negative energies to be transformed into positive ones, to be used for universal goodness.

Reiki Energy Versus Personal Energy

Reiki is a universal source of energy that flows through the practitioner and into the recipient. The practitioner is not giving away any of his or her own energy to the recipient. Nor is the recipient taking energy away from the practitioner.

The fusion of personal energies during treatment can feel as if it is part of Reiki, but that isn't actually the case. The blending of personal energies happens as a consequence of the practitioner and recipient being near each other. Energy fusion experiences can be magnified when individuals empathetically tune in to these personal energies. The personal energy fusion between the practitioner and recipient during a Reiki treatment can be difficult to distinguish from the energy flow of Reiki until you begin to recognize that Reiki has no emotional charge or flavoring.

If Reiki energy were a drink, it would have no taste and could be described as filtered water with no impurities. If personal energies were beverages, they would have distinctive flavors such as sugary colas, pulpy juices, chocolate milk, and so on. You can learn more about empathetically tuning in to personal energies in Chapter 11.

Creating Boundaries

As word spreads within your community that you are a Reiki practitioner, you may find yourself inundated with requests to give Reiki treatments. You may find yourself being asked to give Reiki treatments to your neighbors, relatives, friends, friends of friends, relatives of friends, friends of relatives, and occasionally even pets of your relatives' friends! Yes, you read that right.

It is very important to set clear boundaries and figure out whom you are willing to treat and when you are willing to treat them. You have every right to refuse treatment to anyone without justifying your feelings. Certainly, it is unreasonable to give Reiki to people who you feel are not suitably receptive to it, but it is equally unreasonable for you to feel required to give Reiki every time it is requested of you.

If you ever feel pressured or uneasy when asked to give Reiki to someone, it is a good idea to take some time to evaluate your feelings before agreeing to it. Anytime you feel strongly that you do not want to give a Reiki treatment to someone, embrace those feelings without hesitation and politely refuse.

Dealing with Pushy Requests

One Sunday afternoon a newly attuned Reiki practitioner had a coworker unexpectedly appear at her door with his aging mother in tow. The coworker asked her to treat his mother for her arthritic aches and pains right then and there. This practitioner had offered to share Reiki with this coworker a few weeks earlier, but this was not at all what she had intended. She had not offered to treat her coworker's family member, a woman whom she had never met. Also, having the coworker show up impromptu at her door was ill-mannered, to say the least.

However, the Reiki practitioner felt cornered, and agreed to give Reiki to her coworker's mom so as not to upset either one of them. Needless to say, the impromptu Reiki treatment did not go well. The mother didn't really want to be there and had only agreed to come in order to appease her son. The practitioner felt obliged to help the woman as a favor to her coworker. Neither the practitioner nor the recipient had a clear intent in executing the treatment. Without the unconditional consent of his mother or the practitioner's full readiness, the son's expectation for Reiki to work was unrealistic.

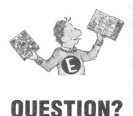

QUESTION?

Are there any limitations to Reiki?
The only limitations that can block Reiki are those we as recipients of the energies set up through a lack of trust or belief in an improved outcome. If our resistance to a cure comes from an unconscious mind, this resistance will limit the flow of ki to bring about complete balance.

This story is just one example of how Reiki, when done under pressured circumstances, is unlikely to result in a positive outcome. It is crucial that the people being treated want the treatment for their own healing journey and not merely to please a friend or relative who thinks they would benefit from Reiki. Question suspected "people pleasers" to ascertain that they are seeking a Reiki treatment for themselves and are not simply trying to appease others. Certainly, the man at the door had good intentions in bringing his mother for treatment. However, until his mother is ready to approach healing on her own terms, Reiki—or any other type of healing modality, for that matter—will be of little use to her and cannot be expected to bring about a significant life change.

It's Up to You

There is no need to get caught up in feelings of inadequacies in giving treatments. You can trust Reiki to deliver to you those people who will benefit from you treating them. However, treating all of them is not mandatory. There will be times when you simply don't feel inclined to work with certain individuals. Be willing to draw a line in the sand. Be firm in your decision not to treat when it comes to giving Reiki treatments to certain people. It may be helpful to know the names and pertinent contact information of other Reiki practitioners in your region to provide as referrals. After all, you are not refusing Reiki to these individuals. You are merely choosing not to serve as the Reiki conduit for them.

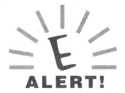

ALERT!

Confidential information about health concerns, relationship difficulties, or family dynamics is often shared between practitioner and recipient. The practitioner should keep all information shared during the session strictly confidential.

Basic Hand Placements for Seniors

Seniors cannot always tolerate a full-body treatment. Nonetheless, they can benefit greatly from frequent shortened sessions. The sessions may be carried out as the recipient is seated in a comfortable straight-backed chair or wheelchair. Before you begin the placements, instruct the recipient to take a few deep, relaxing breaths, and take a few deep, cleansing breaths of your own.

Here are the basic hand placements that may be used for carrying out a shortened Reiki treatment when a person is sitting upright. Hold each position for two to five minutes.

1. **Shoulder Position**—While standing directly behind the recipient, place your hands on both of his shoulders.
2. **Crown Position**—Place your palms on the top of the recipient's head.
3. **Forehead Position**—Move to the recipient's side. Place one hand on the recipient's medulla oblongata, the area between the back of the head and the top of the spine. Place your other hand on his forehead.
4. **Throat Position**—Place one hand on the recipient's seventh protruding cervical vertebra. Place your other hand directly in front of the pit of his throat.
5. **Breastbone Position**—Place one hand on the recipient's breastbone

and the other hand on the recipient's back, in the same area opposite the breastbone.

6. **Stomach Position**—Place one hand on the recipient's solar plexus and the other hand on the back region opposite his solar plexus.
7. **Pelvic Position**—Place one hand on the recipient's front pelvic region and the other hand on the back pelvic region.

Finish the session with an aura sweeping to clear any debris lingering in the auric field of the recipient's body. This should take approximately one minute.

Reiki Treatments at Health Care Facilities

In giving Reiki treatments to patients in hospitals, clinics, and nursing homes, it is important that you do not interfere with any of the facility's rules and routines. Check in with the staff to make sure that your presence and timing of a Reiki treatment for a patient will not interfere with meal times, scheduled lab tests, family visiting hours, and so on.

When paying a home visit, it is helpful to bring along a portable massage table to use during the Reiki treatments. However, bringing along your Reiki table is not usually feasible in hospital rooms, since space is limited and will not accommodate a table.

If the recipient is confined to a hospital bed, do the best you can to apply all the Reiki hand placements. Eliminate any hand placements that you cannot perform easily. If the recipient is not bedfast, you can ask her to sit upright in a bedside chair or lie down in the hospital bed with her head at the foot of the bed in order for you to do the Reiki head placements.

Whether giving Reiki to family members, friends, or clients, giving full-body treatments to others involves time and effort. Reiki will do its job without exhaustion. However, practitioners should remember to honor their own needs first so as not to overspend their personal energies. ⓔ

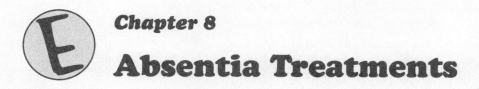

Chapter 8

Absentia Treatments

Absentia Reiki treatments can be given to individuals who are not in physical contact with the Reiki practitioner. Similar to offering prayers, sending Reiki's healing energies remotely involves visualization and mental focus, and it is done as a request for improvement in the recipient's health, life circumstance, and so on. Absentia treatments are not a substitute for hands-on treatments; they are a convenient alternative for circumstances in which it is either impractical or simply not possible to do a hands-on treatment.

The Power of Reiki Symbols

In order to execute remote healing, the Reiki practitioner must rely on the Reiki symbols, which were derived from Japanese kanji characters. Students learn the first three Reiki symbols when they progress to Reiki Level II. It is often the desire to have access to the knowledge and power within these symbols that incites Reiki practitioners to pursue Level II training. Two additional Reiki symbols are learned in Level III. The combined function of these symbols is to give Reiki practitioners focal points for their healing intentions.

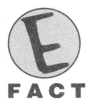

FACT

Reiki symbols are considered sacred and were kept secret for many generations among Reiki practitioners. Even today, many practitioners honor the tradition of keeping them hidden from view by never drawing them on paper and visualizing them from memory alone.

In addition to distant healing, Reiki symbols are used in the attunement process and for directing, focusing, and increasing the flow of Reiki during hands-on healing. Reiki II students are taught how to draw and visualize the Reiki symbols to use in increasing power and focus of hands-on healing. Students are also taught how to use them to send Reiki energies for healing people that are not in their physical presence. These types of treatments are called absentia, remote, or distance healings.

Working with the Symbols

The three Reiki symbols given to Reiki Level II students are the Power symbol, the Connection symbol, and the Harmony symbol. The remaining two symbols, the Master symbol and the Raku, are passed on to the Reiki Level III teacher to utilize in the attunement process when initiating new students to Reiki.

The more you work with the symbols, the more familiar you will become with how each symbol has its own purposes, unique to itself. Learning about Reiki symbols goes far beyond any basic understanding of techniques you could be taught in a class or read in a book. It is through using the symbols when doing self-treatments and giving treatments to others that better understanding will come along. By experimenting with them over a period of time, you will instinctively begin to appreciate how powerfully expansive and fluid these symbols are.

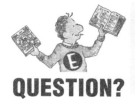

QUESTION?

Why are the Reiki symbols used in absentia treatments? Mental focus is vital to achieving a distance healing. The symbols provide the sender of energy with visual aids for this outcome and also represent intent and empowerment.

The Power Symbol

The first Reiki symbol, Cho Ku Rei, is the Power symbol. It is a spiral-shaped symbol that is often referred to as the Light Switch. The Cho Ku Rei symbol represents the engine that gives Reiki its initial boost. Whenever Reiki needs a nudge to get started or there is a need for an increase in power when applying Reiki, this symbol can be used. In absentia treatments, the Cho Ku Rei serves as the delivery system.

The Harmony Symbol

The second Reiki symbol, Sei Hei Ki, is the Harmony symbol. The Harmony symbol resembles a dragon. Its purpose is to promote the balance and harmony needed to heal our mental and emotional bodies. This symbol is optionally used in absentia treatments.

The Connection Symbol

The third Reiki symbol, Hon Sha Ze Sho Nen, is the Connection symbol. This symbol resembles a pagoda. Its primary purpose is to be used in transmitting absentia treatments. It also serves as a key to unlock information that is kept in the Akashic Records (see Appendix B for a definition of Akashic Records).

Traveling through past, present, and future events, this symbol defies time and space. The Hon Sha Ze Sho Nen is also an excellent tool to use in healings that focus on childhood traumas, inner-child therapy, and past-life issues.

Master and Raku Symbols

The Master symbol, Dai Ko Myo, is utilized in both hands-on and absentia treatments by Reiki practitioners attuned to the Master/Teacher Level. The essence of the Master symbol is love. It is considered the most powerful of all the symbols. The Raku is used only in the attunement process when initiating practitioners into the different levels of Reiki. You can learn more about all of the Reiki symbols in Chapter 16.

The Absentia Healing Formula

The following is a basic formula that utilizes three Reiki symbols used by Reiki Level II practitioners to begin an absentia Reiki treatment. (Reiki Level III Teachers include the Dai Ko Myo symbol in their absentia healing formulas.) This formula has a rhythmic as well as mathematic structure to it.

1. **Draw a Cho Ku Rei symbol for power.** As you draw the Power symbol, repeat the symbol's name three times: Cho Ku Rei, Cho Ku Rei, Cho Ku Rei.
2. **Draw a Hon Sha Ze Sho Nen symbol for connection.** As you draw the Connection symbol, repeat its name three times: Hon Sha Ze Sho Nen, Hon Sha Ze Sho Nen, Hon Sha Ze Sho Nen.
3. **Make your Reiki request.** State your healing intention, including the name and general location of the person to receive the absentia treatment.
4. **Draw a Cho Ku Rei symbol.** As you draw the Power symbol, say it three times: Cho Ku Rei, Cho Ku Rei, Cho Ku Rei.
5. **Draw a Sei Hei Ki symbol for harmony.** As you draw the Harmony symbol, say it three times: Sei Hei Ki, Sei Hei Ki, Sei Hei Ki.
6. **Draw a Cho Ku Rei symbol.** As you draw the Power symbol, say it three times: Cho Ku Rei, Cho Ku Rei, Cho Ku Rei.

Drawing a symbol does not necessarily mean actually drawing it on paper. Although rendering symbols on paper with ink can be very powerful, it is not always practical. You can draw them with your hands in the air and place the air-drawn symbols into objects or draw them mentally by visualizing them in your mind.

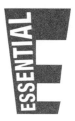

By drawing the symbols, you are bringing them into the open so that they are accessible in the physical world. By exposing them in this way, you are making their potential powers and purposes available to the Reiki recipient.

When drawing symbols in the air to be incorporated in absentia treatments, it is essential that each symbol be drawn completely before it is sent mentally. Symbols sent in fragments will not deliver the highest healing powers that whole symbols will.

Reiki Flash Cards

The absentia healing formula is sometimes taught in a Reiki class through the use of flash cards as instructional aides. Making your own set of Reiki flash cards is fun and easy. Only a few inexpensive materials are needed to make your own: blank index cards, felt-tip marker, a pen or pencil, and one envelope. A complete set of flash cards for sending absentia Reiki to one individual will include:

- Three index cards with the Cho Ku Rei symbol drawn on them
- One index card with the Hon Sha Ze Sho Nen symbol drawn on it
- One index card with the Sei Hei Ki symbol drawn on it
- One blank index card

Use the felt-tip marker to draw the Reiki symbols on the cards. When incorporating flash cards as your focus, you stack the index cards, one on top of another, as you apply the absentia healing formula. Start with a Cho Ku Rei card on the bottom, then place the Hon Sha Ze Sho Nen card on top. Next, using a pen or pencil, write the name of the recipient and your intention statement on a blank index card. Place this request card on top of the Hon Sha Ze Sho Nen card. On top of the request card, you next place the Sei Hei Ki card. Last, place the final Cho Ku Rei card on top of the stack and place all six stacked cards inside a small envelope. Hold the envelope between your hands and allow the Reiki to flow to the recipient. To send Reiki to more than one recipient, simply include another request card and another Cho Ku Rei card for each additional person. As an option, you can include photographs of the recipients along with the Reiki flash cards inside the envelope.

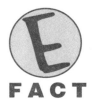

FACT

Using the tongue to draw the Reiki symbols on the roof of your mouth is useful when your hands are busy during a hands-on session. The Cho Ku Rei is the easiest symbol to draw with the tongue.

Directing the Flow

Intention is the means through which Reiki is directed in doing either hands-on or absentia treatments. When giving a hands-on treatment, your primary intention as a practitioner is to facilitate a healing. This intention need not be stated since it is implied when your hands are placed on the body. Reiki will automatically flow to wherever it is needed, with no mental involvement of either the practitioner or the recipient. However, when mental intention is used, a linear pathway is opened. This cleared route allows Reiki to flow more effectively to the part of the body where attention is desired.

Direction is very important when facilitating an absentia healing. Through the use of mental focus, along with the Reiki symbols, Reiki's subtle healing energies can be directed to take a particular path. The practitioner is not *controlling* Reiki by using the symbols and using her mental powers. The practitioner who uses intent is still serving as Reiki's conduit, but with her concentrated involvement, the Reiki will travel more swiftly to the recipient, the main focus of the Reiki energies.

Obtaining Consent

Consent is always a determining factor in giving a Reiki treatment, regardless of whether or not it is carried out in absentia or in person. If your offer to give a hands-on treatment has been rejected, trying to override that person's decision to refuse Reiki by pursuing the route of an absentia treatment would be misguided. Ignoring a person's right to refuse is a deceptive maneuver and could prove damaging to your integrity as a healer.

However, there are a few acceptable circumstances in which you can send Reiki without being given verbal permission by the recipient:

1. The recipient is comatose or is for some other reason incapable of conveying his or her consent.
2. The parent of a young child has requested that you send Reiki to his son or daughter.

Also, there may be occasions when you are asked to send absentia Reiki to someone you are simply unable to contact. An example of this would be when you receive a request to send Reiki to your friend's grandmother's neighbor's uncle who is suffering from an ailment. Getting verbal consent might be possible, but it would require having your friend contact his grandmother, the grandmother contact her neighbor, and the neighbor, in turn, contact the uncle. *Whew!* That could involve a good number of phone calls and the energy of several individuals just to obtain his consent.

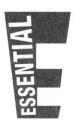

Some people assert that consent is not needed in doing absentia treatments, since a recipient will accept Reiki only if his or her soul-spirit is willing to do so. This opinion seems reasonable and has its merits.

In this type of scenario, consent may be forthcoming, but very time-consuming. Getting consent in this manner can take quite a bit of effort that isn't really expected of the Reiki practitioner. Through the action of the practitioner making an intention statement at the beginning of an absentia treatment, Reiki can easily break through any lack-of-consent barriers.

In Case of Recipient Resistance

It is acceptable for the Reiki practitioner to make an introductory statement of intention in order to indicate that Reiki will become available to the recipient only if he or she is willing to consent to it on a conscious or spiritual level. If you make such a statement, be sure to say that if the recipient declines Reiki, its healing energies will be made available for someone else who is willing to accept them. Some practitioners request that any excess Reiki energies from their absentia sendings be directed to the earth and used for positive global healing.

It is possible for a practitioner who is adept at perceiving the flow of Reiki to feel resistance from the recipient when sending absentia healing energies. Whenever you sense that the Reiki energy is not being welcomed by the recipient, the most appropriate action to take is to discontinue the treatment altogether. Never attempt to force Reiki on anyone who seems inclined to refuse it. To do so suggests that the practitioner is driven by ego, and this is unethical. Never assume that you, as a Reiki practitioner, know what is best for another person.

ALERT!

As an alternative option to drawing the symbols in the air, you can visualize the symbols as designs on rubber stamps that are pressed into an inkpad and then stamped whole into the air.

A More Mindful Approach

For some practitioners, giving an absentia treatment can be inherently more profound than doing a hands-on treatment. This is because possible distractions associated with being in direct contact with the other person's physical body and personality are removed.

When practitioners give hands-on treatments, their perception can be lessened because of people's chatter, masking abilities, body language, and many other factors, thus obstructing a keener awareness. Basically, we are confronted with the storefront dressings of the recipients we treat. Astral connections circumvent any exterior façade that clouds our perceptions when we are in physical contact with others, making our association with them less encumbered with purposeless information.

When you are asked by someone to send absentia Reiki, you are being invited into that person's sacred space. Be respectful during your treatment, since the recipient is making himself or herself vulnerable to your perceptions. This is not the time or place to play the role of an investigator, seeking to discover what secrets might be exposed by psychologically touring the recipient's personal energy field. Be mindful that confidentiality still applies.

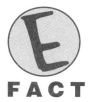

FACT

It is common practice among Reiki practitioners to give an absentia treatment to a person the evening before the scheduled hands-on treatment. Doing this kind of preliminary healing helps ready the recipient's receptivity to Reiki's energies and often predetermines a more profound hands-on healing session.

Absentia Treatment Positions

Absentia Reiki treatments can last as long as full-body hands-on treatments. Find a comfortable chair to sit in while you are giving the distant treatment. An overstuffed chair or recliner works well. During the treatment you will be using your knees, thighs, and hips as spots for placing your hands. To apply the hand placements, imagine a miniature of the recipient lying on his back on your left leg and a miniature of the person lying on his stomach on your right leg. Before you apply your hands, bring forth the Reiki symbols and state your intention as outlined in the absentia healing formula.

Here are the specific hand placements used in absentia treatment:

- Your left knee represents the recipient's face, crown, neck, and jaw line.
- Your left middle-thigh area represents the recipient's heart and upper chest.

- Your left upper-thigh area represents the recipient's ribs and abdomen.
- Your left hip area represents the recipient's pelvic bones.
- Your right knee represents the back of the recipient's head and his neck/throat area.
- Your right middle-thigh area represents the recipient's shoulder blades.
- Your right upper-thigh area represents the recipient's midback and lower-back regions.
- Your right hip area represents the recipient's sacral region.

Apply your hands to these placements on your lap in the same manner that you would give a full-body treatment to a recipient who was actually in your presence. Allow three to five minutes per hand placement.

Teddy Bear Surrogates

A favorite way to send distant Reiki is done by using a teddy bear as a surrogate. Choose a bear that fits comfortably on your lap. With an open hand, draw the Reiki symbols in the air and gently push them with your hand into the head or tummy of the bear as you state your intention for the absentia treatment. Proceed with the Reiki hand placements on the bear in the same manner you would on the recipient if he or she were actually present. You can finish the treatment by hugging the bear as a demonstration of your love being extended to the recipient.

Sending Reiki to a Group

Absentia Reiki can be sent to more than one individual at the same time. The Reiki energies received by the recipients are not lessened as a result of Reiki being dispensed to several people. Each person or group named in the practitioner's intention statement can benefit from the healing energies being offered. You may consider sending Reiki to particular groups of people or even to places or causes:

- Reiki can be sent to general cross-section groups such as farmers, teachers, newborns, firemen, and so on.

- Reiki can be sent to care organizations such as the Red Cross, UNICEF, the Salvation Army, or Habitat for Humanity.
- Reiki can be sent for special causes such as asking for survival of endangered animals, food for the hungry, homes for the homeless, and prosperity for the poor.
- Reiki can be sent to specific health advocate groups such as hospice caregivers, incest victims, and cancer survivors.
- Reiki can be sent to locations such as hospitals, schools, and prisons.

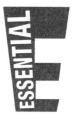

Doing multiple healings clouds the practitioner's perception of how and where the Reiki is flowing. However, it is not always relevant that the practitioner be involved in how the Reiki energy is being used. Serving as a conduit for Reiki to be dispensed for the greater good of all concerned is always gratifying.

Many practitioners make sending absentia Reiki a part of their daily routines, much like a daily meditation practice. They will spend twenty to sixty minutes mindfully sending Reiki out to whoever is in need. You can create a special place in your home where you gather up photographs of people and places, hand-written requests, and names of individuals that you want to include in your absentia sendings. These items can be tacked up on a bulletin board or placed inside a wicker basket, healing box, or family photo album. Ⓔ

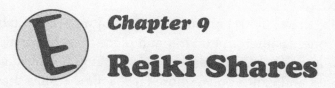

Chapter 9
Reiki Shares

Like-minded individuals naturally congregate to discuss ideas and share their common interests, and Reiki practitioners are no different. They, too, share a fondness for flocking together. It is Reiki's magnetizing love that invokes an impassioned sense of community among its members, drawing them together. Reiki shares offer Reiki practitioners the opportunity to join healing hands in a sacred space. Their combined healing forces not only comfort personal ills but also assist in easing the suffering of all humankind.

Learning to Share

Reiki shares, also known as Reiki circles or Reiki exchanges, are occasions that allow Reiki practitioners to gather together to socialize and participate in group healing treatments. The main purpose for the Reiki share is to give and receive Reiki in a casual atmosphere of friendship, honor, and devotion.

During a Reiki share, the recipient lies down on a massage table while the practitioners gather around her and place their hands upon her, facilitating a massive flow of Reiki energies. Group healings are often very powerful and can produce more far-reaching results than individual healer/client Reiki sessions. Because of the increased flow of many combined hands channeling ki energies, a treatment can be completed in a shortened time period of approximately twenty to twenty-five minutes.

Public Reiki Shares

Everyone is welcome to attend publicly sponsored Reiki shares. These shares are often advertised to draw interest from those members of the general public who know little or nothing about Reiki and who might be curious to learn more.

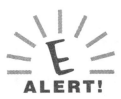

ALERT!

Public Reiki shares are often held in rented rooms, so there may be a modest fee charged to help cover the costs of the healing space used. Do your homework before you attend a Reiki share by phoning ahead to find out if there are any fees or other special requirements.

Public Reiki shares are ideal places for the Reiki practitioners who have not had many opportunities to treat people outside of their immediate circle of friends and family. Often practitioners come to the shares because they have just started working with Reiki and want to get more experience and confidence when giving a treatment.

Finding a Public Reiki Share

Locating publicly sponsored Reiki shares that are open to the general public is not always easy. Because these shares are free or modestly priced, they are not always well advertised. Look for announcements posted on bulletin boards at public libraries, natural-food markets, wellness centers, and metaphysical bookstores.

You can find Reiki share invitations and postings available in your area by doing a search on the Internet. A search engine will quickly provide you with many links to help you find just what you are looking for.

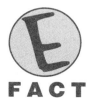

FACT

Smaller tight-knit Reiki communities commonly hold private Reiki shares on a rotation basis, perhaps each week or twice a month. Members take turns hosting shares.

Private Reiki Shares

A private share is an informal gathering of individuals who are attuned to Reiki. These types of shares are generally "invitation only" gatherings and are most often held in a home setting. This type of share offers an opportunity for practitioners to work on each other, learn new techniques, and discuss their experiences in working with Reiki. Because the healers normally know each other on a personal level, private shares are much more relaxed than shares that are open to the public.

Private shares are especially helpful to new initiates, giving them a chance to practice the art of Reiki among seasoned healers. Reiki shares offer a safe haven for you to openly ask questions about giving and receiving Reiki in the company of people who understand what you are talking about.

Hosting a Private Reiki Share

Hosting a Reiki share does not require a lot of work, but, like most events, it would be beneficial for you to do some preliminary planning.

Impromptu shares can be heartfelt as well, but everyone will appreciate the lightness and untroubled atmosphere of a well-organized share.

Taking the time to prepare for your share will make this special healing event more pleasurable for everyone involved. The last thing you want is to be stressed out or exhausted from overplanning this special occasion.

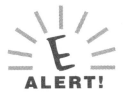

ALERT!

Don't forget to turn off the ringer to your telephone after everyone has arrived so your share will not be disturbed unnecessarily. Ask all the people in attendance to turn off their cell phones.

Choosing a Date and Time

Your first step in arranging a share is deciding the date and time of day to hold your share. Choose the day and time that is most convenient for your own schedule. Your personal comfort level should be your primary concern since everyone attending the share will take his or her cues from you. If you appear frazzled, rushed, or uncomfortable in any way, this will influence the overall climate of your share environment.

Shares may be arranged for mornings, afternoons, or evenings; they generally last between two and four hours, unless they are all-day affairs. Here are a few typical share schedules:

- Morning Reiki share: 8:30 A.M.–12:00 P.M.
- Afternoon Reiki share: 1:00 P.M.–3:30 P.M.
- Evening Reiki share: 7:00 P.M.–10:00 P.M.
- All-day Reiki share: 10:00 A.M.–8:00 P.M.

The time involved in a share depends on how many people are in attendance, how many tables are being used, and how many treatments are applied. Optimally, each guest will have her turn as a recipient of a treatment from the group before the share concludes.

Inviting Your Guests

Invite your guests at least one week prior to your share date. Private shares are routinely very informal affairs, so formal invitations are not necessary. Inviting your guests can be as easy as making phone calls or sending out e-mails. Of course, if you would like to make your share a special event, invitations sent through the mail are quite elegant.

Your personal invitations may include any special requests that you feel are necessary for the success of the Reiki share. Hosts routinely request their guests to bring something along with them to the share—pillows, a fluffy bolster, healthy drinks or snacks, and so on. If you are in need of a massage table, you may ask a guest to tote along her portable table to help you out. If you already have a table but are planning on a large attendance, you might need someone to bring a second table. You should arrange to have one massage table available for every six or seven guests.

Prepare the Healing Space

If you are a Reiki Level II practitioner, you may send future-event/long-distance energies to your event site one day in advance of the share. Add some loving touches to the site as well, in order to make the event feel special. On the day of the share, approximately thirty minutes before your guests are scheduled to arrive, take the time to clear and bless the healing space designated for your share. Here are some suggestions for creating a pleasurable environment for your Reiki share:

- Make certain that the room in which you plan to hold your share is free of dust and clutter. Open the windows to let a welcoming breeze into the room if the weather permits.
- Visualize drawing welcoming Cho-Ku-Rei symbols over the doorways to the room and on the chairs in the space.
- Decorate and harmonize your healing space with feng shui techniques to accentuate your personal tastes. A water fountain gurgling in the background can be a pleasing acoustic touch.

- Having an assortment of colorful and soft pillows scattered about will make everyone feel cozy and pampered.
- Subtly scented incense or aromatherapy candles lit on side tables will enchant the participants of the share.

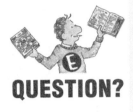

QUESTION?

What is feng shui?
Feng shui (pronounced "fung shway") is the ancient Chinese system of arranging living and work environments through furniture rearrangement, changes in hues and lighting, and the use of plants and decorative objects to maximize harmony, happiness, and well-being.

You can also conduct a ritual sage smudging to dispel any negative or stagnant energies that may be lingering about. The burning of herbs for emotional, psychic, and spiritual purification is common practice among many religious, healing, and spiritual groups. The ritual of smudging can be defined as spiritual house cleaning. In theory, the smoke attaches itself to negative energy and, as the smoke clears, it takes the negative energy with it, releasing it into another dimension where it will be regenerated into positive energy.

Nourishment Planning

It is a good idea to have food and drinks available for everyone to snack on between sessions. Think of simple, healthy food options, and steer away from heavy, sugary, or fatty food choices. Here are a few menu ideas to consider:

- **Breakfast share menu**—Nutritionists agree that breakfast is the most important meal of the day. Fill a cloth-lined wicker basket with an assortment of freshly baked bagels. Offer your guests their choice of peanut butter or strawberry jam for spreading. Orange-carrot juice or apple cider as the beverage will complete your breakfast menu.
- **Afternoon or evening share menu**—For a midafternoon or evening share, try offering lighter fare. Set out small clay bowls filled with

dried cherries, golden raisins, and raw almonds. Brew some chamomile or lemon balm herbal tea for their calming properties.

• **All-day share potluck—**If you are hosting an all-day session, you may opt to prepare a potluck or buffet-style meal. It's a convenient and festive way to share in everyone's favorite foods. You can ask each of the guests to bring along a dish.

In addition, make sure you provide plenty of water. Healers understand the importance of drinking water to flush out toxins, so it is likely that your guests will be equipped with their own bottles of water; nevertheless, it is a good idea to have a supply of bottled water on hand to distribute, just in case.

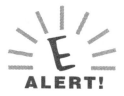

Doing any type of energy work, including Reiki, demands that our bodies have sufficient sustenance to maintain proper energy levels throughout the experience. Fresh or dried fruits, unsalted nuts, bran muffins, low-fat yogurt, fruit juices, green drinks, and herbal teas are excellent nourishment choices.

Setting the Pace

A share group depends on the host to set the pace and flow of the session and treatments. Giving basic instruction to the group will assure that your share functions smoothly.

In order for each person to have his or her turn at receiving Reiki, divide the time allotted to your share by the number of guests to approximate how long your treatments can last. For example, if you have eight guests and your share is scheduled for three hours, you could break the time down to approximately twenty minutes per treatment. This allows two to three minutes between sessions for stretching legs and bathroom breaks. Keep faithful to your schedule and monitor the time for individual treatments with a wristwatch, minute timer, or wall clock. Designate the person sitting at the head position of the Reiki table to keep track of the minutes allowed for each treatment in order to keep everyone on schedule.

Give each person an opportunity to opt out of a session. Sitting out of the session following one's own healing treatment is sometimes needed to help sort out any issues that may have surfaced. Being able to break away from the healing space relieves the pressure of feeling like you need to give back immediately. Having those few minutes for simply relaxing, eating some food, and perhaps sipping on a cup of tea will help bring you back to the present, revive your spirit, and integrate your overall healing processes.

Reiki Share Etiquette

Most healers subscribe to a code of common courtesy and ethical behavior. Shares are held in sacred healing spaces and for this reason it is essential that everyone in attendance demonstrate proper respect. The tone need not be too serious, and it should certainly not be stodgy or rigid. Ideally, the atmosphere of a share is one of friendliness, loving, and cordiality.

Honoring Confidences

Whenever giving Reiki, it is important to honor the healing journey of the recipient. You must keep in confidence everything that's shared during the healing session.

Because of the social and informal setting of a share, it can be difficult to determine what is being said in confidence and what is not. If you have difficulty discerning the difference between a recipient processing deep work and merely sharing an amusing family anecdote, it is better not to repeat any of the discussions outside the confines of the share.

Focus on the Recipient

Experiencing Reiki is sacred and each person participates in it in a different way. As you begin each treatment, attempt to make a heart connection with the recipient, maintaining this connection as your primary focus throughout the allotted session time.

Appreciating Your Host

Honor the host for opening up his or her home and heart in arranging and holding a space for healing. Respect all rules the host has established for the sharing. Some hosts feel it is ill-mannered for anyone to come to a share and not reciprocate fully in the giving and taking of energies. If you are not able to attend the share for the entire scheduled time, you should inform your host in advance to receive permission to leave the session early.

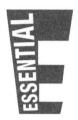

Conversation between the practitioners and the recipient is typical and can make a session feel lighter and easier, but getting caught up in excessive chitchat across the table with other guests while disregarding the recipient's healing process on the table is not appropriate or conducive to a successful healing experience.

Shifting Energies

Don't discount or attribute lesser value to share treatments that are of shorter duration than full-body treatments that typically last an hour or longer. Deep levels of energy work can be accomplished in group healings because of the many hands at work.

You will notice a new and different shift of energy taking place as each person lies down on the table to receive his or her Reiki session. Also, topics of the group's conversation will likely switch from somber to merry and vice versa at the drop of a hat as emotional breakthroughs take place. Because of the empathic nature of many healers, it is not unusual for one or more of them to exhibit emotions that mirror the recipient's experience, such as feeling tearful or melancholy. Keep a box of tissues handy for blowing noses and drying tears of joy and grief.

Shifting of energies during a Reiki share can be quite dramatic and erratic. Imagine taking a six-year-old child to the circus for the first time. The child will be filled with mixed emotions of excitement, chaos, and bewilderment from viewing the clowns, trapeze artists, the fire-eater, and the lion tamer all in one visit. Participating in a Reiki share can be a similarly overwhelming and exhausting experience. This can happen because of the wide range of emotions that are encountered through the different personalities working on their issues. Emotions energetically shared by everyone can range from heartbreak, jubilation, depression, sorrow, sexual tension, rejection, and so on.

Finding a Balance Between Giving and Receiving

Many people have difficulty accepting help or healing. This is especially true of women, particularly mothers, as they are natural givers who don't always know how to receive. Attending shares and allowing yourself to be a receiver of energies will help you find a balance. After attending a few shares and learning to receive, you'll soon be begging to be the first one on the table.

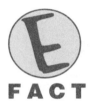

FACT

The Alexandria Reiki Center advocates the practice of tower healing, a concentrated healing on a desired area. Healers stack their hands, one hand on top of another, forming a tower that beams focused Reiki energies toward the needy area.

When the Share Is Over

Experiencing a share can leave you feeling as if you are as sleepy and wobbly as a newborn kitten. Having soaked up so many energies in a short period of time, it can take you quite a while to assimilate everything you have absorbed. It is important that you disengage and neutralize yourself. Go home and take a shower or bath to refresh your relaxed body and restore your spirit. Drink extra amounts of water for the next twenty-four hours. Remember that water is a purifier, both externally and internally. Give in to your needs. If you feel like taking a nap, give in to that feeling. If you are hungry, feed your body. Absolutely take it easy for the remainder of the day.

Pairing Up with a Partner

All Reiki sessions are about sharing—after all, any Reiki practice bestows love to others (or, in the case of self-treatments, to yourself). Reiki shares are group affairs that involve sharing massive amounts of ki energy. Reiki shared from one person to another can also cultivate a significant amount of light and warmth.

Having another person with whom to share Reiki on a regular basis can be a beneficial way to bring balance into your Reiki regimen. Too often, healers give, give, and give some more, without slowing down long enough to take care of their own needs. By pairing up with another Reiki practitioner and routinely taking turns giving and receiving, each of you will begin to notice symmetry and tranquility in your practice of Reiki.

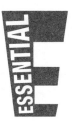

Share communities that gather routinely tend to take advantage of the power of group energy and will sometimes spend a few minutes beaming healing energies to planetary concerns such as weather disturbances (earthquakes, tornados, drought, floods, etc.) and human crises (war, hunger, poverty, etc.).

Reiki shares can be wonderful outlets for practitioners who are reclusive or introspective types, allowing them to participate in the social atmosphere and gain the advantages of sharing Reiki energies. On the other hand, for practitioners who are inclined to be characteristically more social, a discipline of solitary meditation may be needed to create balance. It is through the quiet use of Reiki that intuition flourishes.

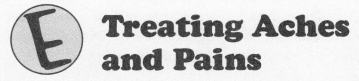

Chapter 10

Treating Aches and Pains

The aches and pains associated with our afflictions are generally our primary concern when we approach treatment. However, our sufferings are much more complex than the dis-eases that afflict the separate components of our physical bodies. In addition to physical discomforts, we suffer from emotional heartbreak and anguish, endure mental stress and anxiety, and struggle with spiritual and moral issues. Reiki addresses those disturbances that are ready to be released or transformed into positive energy.

Treating the PEMS Body

When applying spot treatments for injuries, you touch specific areas with the palms of your hands to facilitate a Reiki healing, and it is especially important to remember that Reiki will naturally flow to wherever it is best suited for each individual. This means that the physical dis-ease may or may not be addressed straight away. Reiki may first treat the recipient's emotional trauma or mental distress before directing its attention to any physical damage. Similarly, Reiki could be blocked from working entirely if the recipient is not at the needed level of acceptance.

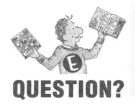

QUESTION?

What does PEMS stand for?
PEMS is an acronym commonly used when referring to our four etheric bodies: physical body, emotional body, mental body, and spiritual body.

Reiki may not immediately heal pains that could be trying to teach us something. This is true with any therapy or healing modality. Our pains teach us to look at our life choices, learned behaviors, or reactions to environmental stimuli, all of which are aspects of life that could possibly need modification. Under these types of life circumstances, Reiki might at first bring about only a release of mental disturbances or emotional flare-ups. This allows the physical manifestation of the dis-ease to linger for a while longer, providing the recipient of the Reiki energy more time to learn tolerance or some other spiritual lesson. Without judgment or expectation on your part, be willing to accept that Reiki flows wherever it is most appropriate and may not affect all parts of your PEMS body.

- **Physical body**—Reiki is applied to our aches and pains as a means of repairing present dis-eases that have affected the muscular and fleshy tissues, internal organs, and blood and bone elements of our physical bodies. Reiki also speeds the recovery time after surgical procedures and offers pain relief from chronic ailments.
- **Emotional body**—Reiki serves as a calming agent and, through its balancing energy, is always ready and able to help disperse and

dissolve feelings associated with emotionally charged situations and relationships. Emotional issues eased by Reiki include feelings of rage, fear, abandonment, rejection, and despair.

- **Mental body**—Reiki offers mental clarity and focus to the confused, distracted, or distraught. Mental distresses such as memory loss, confusion, anxiety, obsessive thoughts, and mania can be placated with the application of Reiki.
- **Spiritual body**—Reiki is a vehicle that allows us to connect more deeply with our spiritual being. As this spiritual connection deepens, we ultimately arrive at a better understanding of the immense potential we have to heal ourselves.

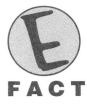

FACT

Reiki is often called "smart" or "intelligent" energy. It knows which areas of the body need healing and automatically flows to those specific sites where suffering or imbalances are prevalent. Reiki will not cause harm to anyone. It is a complementary modality that can be used safely with all other types of treatments.

Bleeding, Broken Bones, and More

Normally, there are two basic rules of thumb when it comes to Reiki treatment:

1. Reiki is an intelligent energy that causes no harm.
2. Placing your hands on the body activates Reiki's healing process.

But in addition to these basic rules, there are also a few important precautions and exceptions to keep in mind when treating certain types of injuries. These injuries are frequently referred to as the First-Aid Bs: bleeding, bumps and bruises, broken bones, burns, and bee stings.

Treating Broken Bones

When treating a broken bone, do not place your hands directly over the break. The concern is that Reiki's swift healing process would be a premature remedy to a twisted, splintered, or misaligned injury. It is okay for you to do Reiki over other parts of the body before the setting has taken place, but wait until after the bone has been properly set before applying Reiki directly over the fracture.

Common sense tells us that repairing a broken bone would require structural manipulation and that an energy modality alone could not reverse the injury. The warning in treating broken bones affirms the perception that Reiki should be considered a complementary therapy alongside other healing modalities, rather than an end-all remedy.

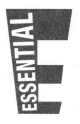

In theory, it could be argued that Reiki is smart enough to reduce only the pain and swelling, refraining from healing the preset bone regardless of where your hands may be positioned. Make your own conclusions with this particular teaching.

Treating Bumps and Bruises

Reiki blocks or diminishes bleeding under the skin upon application. Place your hands directly on your stubbed toes, skinned knees, and other bumped areas until the pain subsides. It is important for Reiki to be applied promptly after injury occurs to block or reduce any bruising.

A Reiki Level I practitioner shared the following story about her own experiences in treating bruises with Reiki. This woman routinely checked into a headache clinic to help the developers evaluate new migraine drugs in hopes of managing and relieving the pain associated with migraines. These test pharmaceuticals were injected intravenously into the veins of both her arms. She was sensitive to the needle pokes and would return home with black-and-blue marks up and down both arms. After receiving her Reiki I attunement, she decided to test Reiki's effect on bruising during her next visit to the clinic. She applied Reiki to one of her arms, leaving the other one untreated. She happily reported the results of her experiment. The bruising was minimal on the arm she treated with Reiki, whereas her other arm exhibited unsightly purple streaking and black-and-blue bruising.

Treating Burns and Sunburns

When applying Reiki to burned skin, don't touch it directly. Instead, allow your hands to hover over the burned area at a comfortable distance. There are several reasons for why you should avoid touching the skin. First of all, it's important to safeguard against possible infection to the burned area. Burns are susceptible to infection, and touching invites undesirable contaminants that may further complicate or interfere with the healing process. The second reason is that Reiki energies often generate beaming rays of hot energy. These penetrating streams of hot energy could bring about additional pain or discomfort to the burn victim.

Remember, Reiki energies and symbols can be placed into anything to assist healing and transformation. In treating sunburns you can put healing Reiki rays into aloe vera gel by either holding the bottle between your hands before applying it to the skin or by beaming energies into the gel as it is being distributed to the wound. To protect your skin from the elements, such as dry air and scorching sunrays, you can place Reiki's Protection symbol, Sei Hei Kei, into sun-block lotions and moisturizing creams.

Treating Bleeding Injuries

Precautions cited in caring for bleeding wounds are similar to those suggested in treating burns. Do not touch areas that are bleeding, because, in doing so, you could expose the area to possible infections. Also, it is especially important to be careful when treating anyone who is bleeding because of the possible transfer of blood-borne pathogens, like HIV and hepatitis B.

Treating open cuts and injuries with Reiki to slow or stop the flow of blood is helpful. Actually, Reiki will likely begin to take effect without any intent on your part as you apply pressure on a bloody wound to manage the blood flow. In treating minor cuts, don't be too concerned about stopping the bleeding immediately, since initial bleeding can help cleanse a cut wound of any fragments of metal, glass, or rust that may have become deposited into the wound by the cutting implement. After the injury has been properly cleaned and bandaged, applying hands-on spot treatment will help hasten restoration.

Treating Bee Stings

In applying immediate spot treatment to relieve yourself of the painful burning sensation from a bee sting, carefully cup or arch your hands over the sensitive area of the body. Be careful not to touch the stung area directly, since this may result in burying the animal's stinger more deeply into the flesh, making it difficult to extract later and possibly leading to an infection. Remove the stinger with sterile tweezers, either before or following the Reiki treatment.

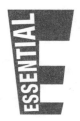

The common plantain, a weed plant, can help relieve the pain and distress associated with bee stings. In the Old World, plantain is also a common remedy for cuts, sores, burns, snake and insect bites, and inflammations. This weed should not be confused with the type of banana that bears the same name.

Heartburn and Indigestion

Our digestive systems don't always tolerate the foods that entice our palates. When we overindulge, we can become victims of heartburn, indigestion, nausea, or stomach cramps. Fortunately, the gentle and calming effect of Reiki's energetic flow may ease internal discomforts such as heartburn and upset stomach.

You can quickly neutralize gastric flare-ups by placing your hands upon the chest or abdominal area. Taking a few deep breaths during application will help Reiki break through internal blockages. A good habit to develop is blessing your meals with Reiki before ingestion in order to stave off potential stomach problems.

Treating Hard-to-Reach Areas

Applying hands-on Reiki to certain areas of our bodies for more than a brief period can make one feel like a pretzel and lead to uncomfortable cramping or stiffness in the process. Doing so would not be a problem if you were a trained gymnast or student of Yoga, accustomed to bending, stretching, and folding your body in a variety of positions. But for most people, the discomfort of keeping hands placed on certain areas of our bodies for a prolonged period of time can prove burdensome. How many minutes would you be comfortable bent over while keeping your hands on your feet to treat a bunion?

Being attuned to Level II of Reiki can come in quite handy. When treating hard-to-reach places, Reiki II practitioners can direct energies into their teddy bear surrogates to be sent to the awkward location (see Chapter 8 for more on distance treatments). Hemorrhoids can be treated successfully by placing your hands on the backside of your surrogate teddy bear while intentionally beaming warm vibes and healing energies to be transferred to your sore, swollen tissues.

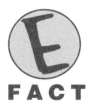

FACT

In Chinese medicine, the meridian healing system is based on the concept that an insufficient supply of ki (chi) makes a person vulnerable to disease. Restoring the ki is the ultimate goal in restoring overall health and well-being to the individual. Acupuncturists, Chinese herbalists, massage therapists, and Reiki practitioners utilize their various healing methods to assist clients in repairing dysfunctional areas to restore a natural balance.

Anxiety and Phobias

Reiki is a practical remedy for calming our fears and reducing anxiety. Even if you are not ordinarily a Nervous Nelly type, relying on Reiki as a calming agent is a good idea. Everyone experiences anxious moments and/or traumatic situations that can create confusion, excitability, or even force you to just freeze in your tracks. With the help of Reiki, you may be able to overcome certain phobias, like the fear of of public speaking, death, flying, hospitals, darkness, water, heights, poverty, thunderstorms, or riding in elevators.

Being equipped with Reiki is like having someone next to you at all times of day and night to hold your hand and help guide you through the occasional rough patches you encounter in your daily life. There is no longer any need to scramble about, looking for a plain brown paper bag to breathe into whenever you feel you might be hyperventilating. Reiki is available 24/7. No matter what type of situation you are facing when fear grips you, Reiki is at your side to help alleviate overcharged energies by bringing in a lower vibration to create a calmer state of mind.

During the course of a day, we often find ourselves confronted with situations that frustrate or upset us. Rather than giving in to feelings of impatience when you are caught in heavy traffic and are in a hurry, try placing your hands on yourself and let Reiki bring you some peace and tranquility. Take advantage of any occasions during your daily routine, whether you're standing in line at the supermarket checkout or sitting in the waiting room before a doctor appointment, to give yourself a Reiki "booster shot." You'll be pleasantly surprised at how quickly any feelings of impatience or frustration will diminish or become dispelled entirely after you allow Reiki to come to your emotional rescue.

For Chronic Pain Sufferers

Chronic pain sufferers consistently seek out new healing modalities to help them manage their dis-eases and discomforts, and for this reason may choose to give Reiki a try. In treating others with chronic pain it is especially important not to tout Reiki as a cure-all but rather to emphasize that it functions efficiently when used for pain management. There are no quick fixes in applying Reiki to conditions that are identified as chronic. Reiki should be considered a complementary remedy that can safely be used in conjunction with other therapies to assist in healing processes.

Using Prescription Drugs

Reiki can be phenomenally effective when applied as a pain manager. After experiencing the pain-numbing effects of receiving consistent Reiki treatments, you might feel like tossing out any pain medications prescribed by your doctor. Never stop taking any prescribed drugs without the supervision of your physician. When certain medications are suddenly stopped altogether, complications may occur. Communicate to your health care providers that you are using Reiki to help manage your pain. Let them know that you are receiving Reiki treatments and that you believe you are feeling better because of them. You might also request that your physician re-evaluate any medications that you are presently using. Taking fewer dosages, reducing their strength, or discontinuing certain prescription drugs entirely may be indicated for your improved condition.

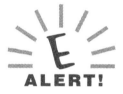

ALERT!

When it comes to pain management and treatment of chronic pain, it is recommended that you undergo consistent and regularly scheduled full-body Reiki sessions. Reiki can help alleviate the pain, stresses, and agitations that are associated with long-term suffering.

Surgical Procedures

Incorporating the use of Reiki in your treatment plan when surgery is in the picture will help this intrusive procedure feel less traumatic. Some people have reported that using Reiki resulted in less pain, minimal blood loss during the surgery, and shortened recovery period.

Prior to surgery, a series of preop Reiki treatments can be given to prepare and comfort the body from the trauma of being surgically cut and to support the body's own healing processes that will naturally follow. You can also send future-event/long-distance energies prior to the time of the scheduled surgery.

During the operation, a Reiki practitioner can send absentia Reiki to the surgical patient. This can be done from nearby, like from the waiting room at the hospital where the surgery is being done, or from far away. In addition, the patient may prepare a healing gemstone charged with Reiki energies and tape it to the palm of his hand, where it would remain throughout the operation.

Just after the operation, the patient may receive a postop Reiki treatment in the recovery room. He should continue to receive postop Reiki treatments daily for as long as needed to hasten the recovery period.

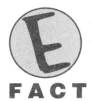

FACT

Coming to terms with death isn't easy. Reiki has successfully made its debut into the hospice arena, allowing Reiki practitioners to assist the dying during the final days of their lives.

Living with Terminal Illness

Fighting a terminal illness takes a lot of energy out of a person. Reiki can help replenish lost energy to help in the battle for a better quality of life.

Treating someone with a dreadful dis-ease such as cancer is an act of love that cannot be measured. It takes a special person to be able to care for someone who is looking death in the face. As the facilitator of Reiki, channeling large quantities of Reiki energy can be draining, so teaming up with a group of healers for a healing session is worth considering.

If you are the sole healer, please remember to take care of your needs first. You will not be doing anyone any favors by wearing yourself out. Rather than giving a full treatment in one sitting that would likely involve one or more hours of constant Reiki flow, break the session into fifteen-minute sequences, allowing yourself five to ten minutes of rest between the shorter sessions.

Transformative Energy

Reiki, much like prayer, is a personal exercise that can easily convert negative energy into positive energy. For this reason, Reiki is truly a profound and transformative healing experience that can be used to assist a person's transitional journey from the physical earth to that of the spiritual realm. Reiki has also been recognized for the great comfort it offers to the family members and loved ones of someone who is in his or her final days or who has already passed on.

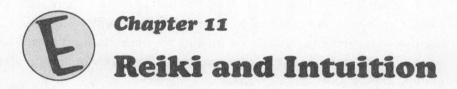

Chapter 11

Reiki and Intuition

Intuition plays a major role in the application of Reiki, even though the spiritual component of this healing art is more apparent to some than to others. During Reiki sessions, most practitioners and recipients notice at least some vibrational shifts of energy. Because the source of Reiki's energies is a universal powerhouse, using this energy opens the participants to experiencing deeper aspects of themselves. These spiritual experiences can range from noticing subtle cues to realizing awesome inspirations.

Connecting with Your Guides

Nothing written in this book is designed to convince anyone to change his or her beliefs. Reiki works whether you believe in it or not—and whether or not you believe in angels, spirit guides, God, Allah, or any other spiritual being or deity.

Holding a belief in spirit guides and such is not a requirement for Reiki. However, it is important to note that the majority of people who are drawn to Reiki as a hands-on healing art often do tend to be spiritually oriented or religious in some way. They may believe in spirit guides, angels, God, or other deities.

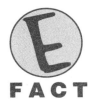

FACT

Some people will speak of connecting with new healing energies after becoming attuned to Reiki or having worked regularly with Reiki. They often attribute these energies to spiritual helpers or Reiki guides.

Communicating with Higher Aspects

Everyone has the ability to communicate with "higher aspects" of himself or herself, with or without using Reiki. Higher aspects represent whatever higher power you are aligned with: God, angels, animal totems, spirit guides, higher self, soul-body, heart center, inner dialogue, and so on.

The attunement process that takes place in Reiki classes clears away blockages in the physical body, helping these loftier types of communications to occur more easily. Through continued use of Reiki, the passageways in your body through which the ki energies flow will frequently be flushed of newly acquired debris and will consequently be broadened. This cleared and broadened passageway is a direct communication avenue, similar to a "pipeline" or "telegraph wire," that provides people with a stronger awareness of their spiritual components, such as the Reiki guides.

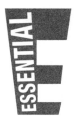

Reiki guides may be described as healing specialists. In much the same way as muses are said to inspire artists and musicians throughout the creative process, Reiki guides influence healers when they are practicing the healing arts.

Reiki guides provide practitioners with the information needed to assist them in applying Reiki treatments. As the Reiki practitioner further develops his intuitive abilities, the Reiki guides orchestrate the healing sessions more and more in order to allow the healing energies to operate with greater fluidity. They direct where the Reiki practitioner's hands need to be placed on the recipient's body and when the hand placements should be changed. Finally, they suggest what kinds of questions to ask the recipient to further assist the practitioner in conducting a proper and thorough Reiki treatment. It is through this guidance that a practitioner is able to connect with the "soul-body" of his recipient and more fully support the recipient in her healing journey.

The Promise of Reiki Guides

Diane Stein was introduced to her personal Reiki guides while doing healing work as a Reiki Level II practitioner. She wrote about this experience in her book *Essential Reiki: A Complete Guide to an Ancient Healing Art*. In the same book, Stein also described how many of her students became aware of their own personal Reiki guides after only a few months of working as Reiki II practitioners. Finding their Reiki guides through practice of Level II Reiki seemed to her a shared experience among all of her students.

Essential Reiki has been widely published and was the introduction to Reiki for many people when it first went into print in 1995. It soon became something like an urban legend to assume that all Reiki Level II practitioners would "meet their guides." Some Reiki II classes are still promoted with the assurance that the students will meet their Reiki guides as a part of the class curriculum. Some teachers even lead guided meditations, inviting the Reiki guides to join their class sessions.

False Expectations

As a result, some students sign up for Reiki classes not so much to learn the healing art but to have the opportunity to be attuned and miraculously be connected with their guides. Naturally, those students who are not able to instantly "see" or "hear" their guides become disappointed. Frustrations are compounded when other Reiki initiates share personal stories of their own guide connections during the class sessions. The students who do not forge a connection with their Reiki guides assume that there is something wrong with them or that the Reiki attunement didn't work.

The disappointment experienced by some of these students is unfortunate. Diane Stein never stated or implied in her writings that all Reiki Level II students must experience meeting their Reiki guides. High expectations of events that never bore fruit were simply the result of information that was taken out of context. Stein wrote of her own experiences in working with Reiki. She never spoke of the awareness of healing guides as something that happens spontaneously. Yet, somehow an expectation grew out of her writings about Reiki guides that prompted some individuals to seek out Reiki in the first place. Many of these people might not otherwise have done so.

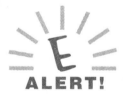
ALERT!

Our expectations in life are often what trip us up. This is especially true when you pair expectation with Reiki. It is best to approach Reiki with no expectation and allow your personal experience with it to unfold naturally.

Paying Attention to the Signs

Those who do make contact with Reiki guides don't necessarily have a visual connection. Ideally, it is best to move beyond the perception that Reiki guides have to be visualized. You don't have to "see" angels or spirit guides in order to prove that you are spiritually aware or that you have accessed inner knowledge. Not everyone acquires spiritual guidance visually.

It is important to pay attention to extrasensory spiritual messages. When we neglect to notice the simpler messages conveyed by a spirit that needs our attention, these communications will eventually be demonstrated in more recognizable ways that you may not appreciate.

Pay attention to subtle nuances. Train your intuition to become aware of messages conveyed by a spiritual source. Listen with your heart—within it, there is a storehouse of wisdom at your disposal that you can tap into at any time, any place. Staying in close communication with your inner dialogue will assist you in making choices that will ultimately affect your life in positive ways.

Listening to Your Inner Dialogue

Most of us make listening to our inner guidance more difficult than it needs to be. We allow our expectations to mirror the experiences that others have described to us. Each of us is unique in the ways we intuit information. Learning how to quiet yourself and tune in to your inner dialogues takes some practice, but the goal is realizable. Allow your expectations to melt away. Figuratively speaking, lean your ear against your heart and listen intently. Here are a few suggestions for flexing your intuition muscles:

- Expand your intuitive ear by quieting your physical ears. Turn off your radio, stereo, and television. Spend a half-hour each day in quiet meditation or solitude.
- Go for a nature walk by yourself. Allow your psyche to merge with sounds of the forest, seashore, mountain trail, etc.
- Pay attention to energy shifts in your physical body. Pain is a signifier that something is wrong.
- Keep a dream journal. Dreams are one of the easiest avenues through which intuitive messages are filtered.
- Take a moment every day to clear away unproductive thoughts and to release cerebral distractions and obsessive mental chatter. Visualizing a chalkboard being erased of these thoughts can be a helpful exercise.
- Keep a synchronicity diary to write down all the "coincidences" you experience throughout the day. Remember, there is no such thing as a coincidence!

- Follow your hunches. Prepare to be amazed where they lead you.
- Pay attention to what emotions or memories are invoked when you are around specific scents.
- Start noticing markers or signs that bring about particular sensations in your gut.

Try not to get overly preoccupied with figuring out the reasons for every little thing that happens in your daily life. When you begin to perceive messages that you don't fully understand right away, just remind yourself that it is not always necessary to know the full meanings of these messages. Explanations tend to come along with intuitive messages on a "need to know" basis. Using your sixth sense is just like flexing a muscle. It will get stronger the more you exercise it.

Emotional Centers of the Body

The strongest "feeling centers" in the body are the heart and the solar plexus region. Our heart-felt emotions originate in the heart. This is the place from which our love of self and love for others flows. This is also the area where our emotional hurts and wounds are stored.

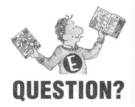

QUESTION?

What is the "solar plexus"?
Your solar plexus is located at the pit of your stomach. It consists of a dense cluster of nerve cells and supporting tissue and is located behind the stomach, directly below the diaphragm. The solar plexus is the area of the third vortex within the seven-chakra system.

In Touch with Your Heart

There is no right or wrong feeling that comes from the heart. These feelings are what they are, pure and simple. No shame or blame should be placed upon anyone because of the way he or she feels—whether it's love or hate, humility or anger, happiness or sadness, guilt or grief, calm or fear and anxiety. Acknowledging one's feelings without judgment is the first step toward healing heart wounds.

Learning forgiveness, trust, unconditional love, and compassion are spiritual challenges associated with the heart region. Emotional empowerment can be achieved by releasing repressed negative feelings that shadow our purest and most positive emotions.

A heart-to-heart communication can be intuited while giving a Reiki treatment. The following exercise can be an overwhelming emotional experience for the practitioner because of the outpouring of love that is transferred from the recipient's heart into the practitioner's. The outcome can be quite profound.

A Heart-to-Heart Exercise

While applying the throat and heart hand placements on the recipient's body, focus on your own heart. Visualize your heart chakra spinning in a clockwise motion. While it continues to spin, shift your focus to the recipient's heart and visualize his or her heart chakra spinning in a clockwise motion as well. Imagine both heart chakras spinning in unison and connecting with one another.

Open your heart and listen for any messages that are intuitively conveyed. Pay close attention to the messages, as if you are a parent listening to your beloved son or daughter, keeping any information received strictly confidential. Silently acknowledge that you totally accept the recipient just as he or she is. From your heart, extend your unconditional love to the recipient.

On a Hunch

Our inner knowledge originates in the solar plexus. This region of the body defines our self-esteem and personal power. Strong self-esteem is a requirement for developing intuitive skills. When we choose to ignore our gut instincts, we are only hurting ourselves further by distrusting messages that are meant to help us. The more often we allow ourselves to follow the direction of our gut feelings, the clearer the intuitive pathway will become. By following through on everyday hunches, no matter how unimportant they may seem, we are actually taking test drives, virtually honing our listening skills.

Trusting Your Feelings

The most frustrating thing about receiving information from a spiritual source is that it often comes through in such a way that you can't make sense of it right away. It is as if the message is written in a foreign language or secret code, and yet you must try to read and comprehend it. Not only that, but there is no translator present to help you crack the code or understand the message.

Interpreting these confusing messages can be quite challenging. Generally, the analytical brain wants to jump in and decipher the messages, but this often creates more confusion. Dissecting the messages with methodical reasoning can prove interesting, but it isn't always helpful. Doing this removes you even further from your emotional body.

To interpret intuitive messages, you need to process them with your emotional body rather than your mental faculties. What feeling did the message invoke in you? Sadness? Happiness? Loneliness? Confusion? Did it bring up repressed feelings from an unresolved issue? Once you can identify the "feeling," you will have something to work with.

Emotional Release

A Reiki treatment is often the trigger that elicits messages to help a person get in touch with the feelings that need to be expressed. By invoking the Hon Sha Ze Sho Nen symbol, you can direct Reiki to delve deeper into any feelings that have surfaced from within the recipient.

Occasionally a person will experience an intense emotional release during or after a Reiki treatment. These types of emotional releases may be expressed through crying, screaming, coughing, or even vomiting. Emotional releases help carry the person through the hurts and discomforts associated with the feelings that arise during a Reiki session.

Sharing Communication

When you intuit messages from your Reiki guides concerning the recipient you are treating, it is up to you to decide whether or not to pass on these messages to the recipient. Trust your feelings in making these decisions. Sometimes the guides provide the practitioner with particular information during a treatment in order to assist him or her in the healing itself. At other times, the guides intend the messages to be shared with the recipient.

A medical intuitive is a psychic or intuitive counselor who specializes in perceiving information concerning the human body. Medical intuitives will intuitively scan a person's body, looking for imbalances that need alignment or treatment.

Sometimes the information that comes through will not make sense to you. In this case you might be inclined to disregard it. However, oftentimes the message will have a feeling of urgency or persistence attached to it. If this is the case, it is likely the message needs to be shared with the recipient. Although the message might not make sense to you, it might actually have a special meaning to the recipient. The message can be subtle, but if it keeps surfacing again and again, don't ignore it. There are also occasions when the recipient is not open to receiving intuited information directly, and the practitioner will serve as a channel through which a recipient's spirit guides can pass on communications.

Are You an Empath?

Natural empaths are individuals who feel the emotions and physical ailments of the people around them. As children, empaths are often called "overly sensitive" because their feelings are easily hurt and they have difficulty controlling their emotions. As a defense mechanism, many empathic children quickly learn to shield themselves from absorbing other people's emotions. As empathic children become adults, it can be a challenge for them to lower their protective walls in order to form loving relationships, rather than isolating themselves from everyone around them.

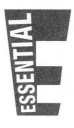

Traits of a natural empathy include sensitivity, compassion, good listening skills, a need to serve as a peacemaker to others, a strong sense of caution, and a quiet, guarded disposition.

Empathy As a Healing Tool

Among healers, the gift of empathy can be a wonderful healing tool, as long as it is used cautiously. It doesn't matter whether you've had this gift since childhood. Empathetic awareness is often acquired and further developed by practitioners as they continually practice Reiki. Used as an awareness tool for intuiting illness and dis-ease, empathy can offer information relevant to those problems that challenge the recipient. Reiki practitioners who are empaths use the intuited information to assist them in their hand placements and in directing the flow of Reiki.

It is important that the practitioner be able to discern the difference between feeling the recipient's ailments and experiencing his or her own health issues. When an empathic practitioner feels general discomforts during a treatment, it's a good idea to consult with the recipient by asking her how she feels. For example, if you get a cramp in your leg or suddenly feel nauseated, ask the recipient if she is experiencing the discomfort as well. After you realize that a pain or discomfort you are experiencing doesn't belong, release it as quickly as possible. Do not continue to hold on to it.

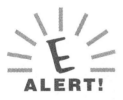

Although empaths "feel" the pain, they do not actually take it away from others. An empath merely intuits information with regards to how the other person is feeling. In shamanic healing methods, the shaman will take the client's issues and physical problems into his or her body for transmutation and transformation. This specialized healing technique should not be used without extensive training.

Releasing Empathized Illnesses

Taking on the illness itself in order to better understand the recipient's state of health is invaluable. However, it is essential not to hold those energies in your body any longer than necessary. Acknowledge the empathized information that was offered, silently thank your spirit source for the knowledge its guidance has offered you, and ask that the discomfort be released from your body.

Allow the discomfort to fade away as you continue treating the recipient. If the "empathized feeling" does not subside and your discomfort continues, you may need to disconnect from the recipient for a few seconds by removing your hands from his body. In severe cases, you may need to discontinue the treatment altogether.

Empathic Reiki practitioners can be conflicted between wanting to intuit feelings in order to use them as a source of knowledge for treating someone and not wanting to feel the discomfort. For these individuals it is best that they shield themselves entirely from taking on illnesses. The Reiki Protection symbol, Sei He Kei, can be utilized to assist them in creating protective walls between them and the people they treat. Allowing yourself to take on others' illnesses is putting yourself at risk until you have learned how to either shield yourself or become accomplished at quickly releasing these ills and discomforts.

Transmuting Negative Energies

Reiki treatments often cause emotional and mental issues that might have become trapped or buried in the recipient's body to surface. This offers an opportunity for any negative and stagnant energies to move upward and outward.

Because these energies are damaged and contaminated, it is cleansing and healing to have them lifted out of the body. However, it is important that these energies be transmuted and transformed into positive energy before they are allowed to re-enter the universe, where they might inadvertently "infect" someone else. If you have ever walked into an empty room and felt a negative emotional charge (we may call these negative charges "bad vibes"), you have experienced what it is like to suddenly come upon discharged energy that has not been transmuted. Leaving discharged negative energy out in the open for others to stumble over is equivalent to leaving smelly garbage out on your street or dumping your dirty laundry for others to trip over.

Clear the "Aura-Ways"

During the treatment, anytime you feel discharged energy accumulating, take a moment to energetically clear the auric field by sweeping it away to be transmuted. Some healers will send these energies to the "white light" to be purified and transformed.

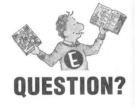

QUESTION?

What is white light?
White light is the space within the universe that is filled with positive energies. White light can be used only for good purposes and can be called upon for protection from negative energies. It can neither come to harm nor cause harm. When anything is sent to the white light, it is balanced and charged with positive energy.

Always conclude a full-body treatment by combing the recipient's aura to clear it of any energetic debris that has lifted from the physical body during the treatment. To do this, move your hands in multiple circular motions or in feathering sweeps over the recipient's body. As you sweep away the debris, you may want to make a prayerful request for the negative energies to be transmuted and transformed into positive energies to be used for universal goodness. It is also recommended that you clear your healing space between Reiki treatments so that there are no lingering energies that could interfere with the healing process of the next Reiki recipient.

Channeling Spirits

In essence, whenever you receive any type of spiritual communication, it is considered a form of channeling. However, the term *channeling* normally means that a person is being used as a human loudspeaker to communicate information from a particular spirit that wants to convey a message to one or more people and sometimes to the world at large.

There are two types of spirit channeling—trance channeling and conscious channeling. Trance channelers are able to set aside their conscious selves in order to loan their bodies for communication with another energy form. These energy forms have many names: spirit guides, spirit entities, Ascended Masters, and so on. Conscious channelers do not give up their conscious selves entirely when they allow information to be channeled through them. Communications that are the result of conscious channeling will have a certain percentage of distortion because it is censored to some degree by the channeler's personality.

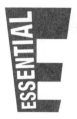

Reiki healing is a form of channeling, but rather than serving as a megaphone or loudspeaker through which words are projected in channeled communications, the Reiki practitioner is more like a pipeline or conduit through which healing energies are transferred.

The more common conscious channelers and the much less common trance channelers could easily be classified as skilled psychics. Depending on their fields of expertise, psychic specialists will refer to themselves with such labels as medium, spiritualist, and medical intuitive. Here is a short list of the most famous channelers of the past and present:

- Alice A. Baily, occult teacher
- Caroline Myss, medical intuitive
- Donald Neal Walsch, conversed with God
- Edgar Cayce, the Sleeping Prophet and founder of the Association for Research and Enlightenment
- James Van Praagh, medium
- Jane Roberts, trance channeler
- John Edward, medium
- J. Z. Knight, Ramtha, or the Enlightened One
- Paula Muran, medical intuitive
- Sylvia Browne, medium

During the Reiki attunement process, the avenue that is opened within the body to allow Reiki to flow through also opens up the psychic communication centers. This is why many Reiki practitioners report having verbalized channeled communications with the spirit world. In some cases, practitioners claim to have received additional information regarding the Reiki system through their channeling. You can read more about channeling Reiki in Chapter 1.

A Spiritual Quest

The Reiki devotee often will dedicate much of her life to spiritual pursuits, including introspection and exploring intuition. Many a seeker has stumbled across Reiki while making her journey through life. Reiki, along with its principles, is quickly accepted as a "valuable find" that assists anyone who wants to continue along the pathway toward well-being and self-discovery. Many people, after engulfing themselves in the teachings of Reiki, will adopt Reiki as their ultimate way of life.

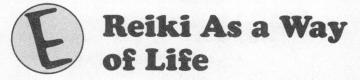

Chapter 12

Reiki As a Way of Life

The Reiki practitioner who embraces all of Reiki's principles and conducts healings on a regular basis will most likely enjoy a more fulfilling life than he or she would otherwise enjoy. Reiki can be integrated into all aspects of your daily life to assist you in meeting your goals and to help you deal with any problems that arise. You can call upon Reiki's stress-reducing energies whenever you are confronted with episodes of anxiety, adversity, or affliction in your everyday life.

A Part of Your Every Day

Our lives are filled with daily rituals. Many people don't think of themselves as being ritualistic because they do not belong to any religious organization or group. Perhaps you do not cast Wiccan spells, participate in Native American peyote rituals, perform Jewish folk dances, or visit the mosque to say your daily prayers. However, this does not mean that you are not ritualistic.

Human beings are habitual animals. Our habits may not feel like rituals because they are not necessarily influenced by a particular religion, dogma, or spiritual belief, but they are rituals nonetheless. We get comfortable with our routines and repeat them again and again. Almost every day we crawl out of bed, bathe, groom, and clothe our bodies, read our newspapers, drive to work or walk to school, eat the customary three meals, work out at the gym, and perform many other routine activities, all at regular repeated time intervals. Re-enacting these daily routines is the equivalent of performing a ritual.

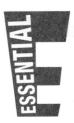

Using Reiki regularly does not mean that your life will always operate perfectly. You will still face challenges, because this is how human life is designed. The difference is that with Reiki, the hurdles won't seem as high and life struggles won't be quite as harsh.

Adjustment and Integration

When we lose an hour of sleep or skip a meal, our bodies react to the change by feeling tired or hungry. Although some people are more flexible and will adjust to change more readily, most of us are to some degree resistant to accepting changes. A common question that students will ask in a Reiki class is "How can I squeeze a daily full-body Reiki treatment into my already hectic twenty-four-hour day?" Already these students are wondering how Reiki will fit into their world without upsetting their comfortable routines. The answer: adjustment and integration.

New parents will anxiously prepare a nursery to make room for the arrival of a new baby into their family. Bringing home the newborn can dramatically change the dynamics of the once childless domicile. The parents are now faced with night feedings, diaper changes, the baby's crying, and so much more. However, after a while, both parents will modify their routines to accommodate their new family member. In a few short weeks, the couple cannot imagine their lives without the child. They love their new baby and are more than willing to accept the changes that parenting requires in order to reap the full benefits of being parents.

There May Be Dramatic or Subtle Changes

Inviting Reiki into your life is much like welcoming a new baby into your family. At first, the introduction of Reiki energies within your body will likely upset your routines. You may find yourself losing sleep or you may discover that you need more sleep than normal. A change in sleeping patterns is simply one possible consequence of being a Reiki practitioner.

Reiki treats imbalances in the body to bring about overall good health and well-being. If your body is lacking in sleep, diet, exercise, or something else, Reiki energies will accordingly cause drowsiness, stimulate food cravings, or promote the desire for you to start pumping iron or find another form of exercise. These changes start to take place at the onset of the Reiki attunement process. For some people, routines will change drastically; for others, there will be only a slight change. How dramatic or subtle the changes will depend on the degree of balancing that needs to be reached in order to create level and calm energies within each person.

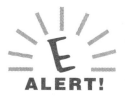

Reiki attunements and Reiki treatments can initially bring about major shifts in your body in order to bring balance. Common changes people have reported are changes in sleep patterns, food cravings, laughter, sexual desire, bowel movements, and weight.

As you continue to practice Reiki, your routines will shift as needed and eventually stabilize to a "new normal" that is appropriate for you. These changes will occur less erratically the longer you practice Reiki on a regular basis. Your body will learn to adjust to these shifts and welcome the relief Reiki offers in aligning your energies on a regular basis. Whenever you feel sick or tense, rather than telling yourself to "chill out" or reaching for that bottle of pain-relief pills, simply place your hands on your body to allow calm and peace to equalize your upsets.

On Rocky Relationships

It is ill-advised for a Reiki practitioner to treat an emotionally close person during a period when their relationship has become strained or problematic. This advice applies to *any* personal relationship that turns less than amicable. It makes no difference whether the person in question is your spouse, lover, sibling, parent, child, friend, or neighbor. Do not give them Reiki until the relationship has been mended.

Giving a Reiki treatment is not recommended at these times because the practitioner may have an underlying ego-involvement or emotional block that could interfere with the healing process—whether or not the practitioner is aware of it. Also, it is likely that the recipient would resist any offer of Reiki from the individual because of the unfriendly status of their relationship. It is best to wait until the problem has been resolved and the relationship has returned to its normal closeness; then, you can both feel fully open to conduct another Reiki hands-on treatment.

Over Distance

One way of dealing with the problem is for the practitioner to send Reiki directly to the troubled relationship by using the distant formula. In this type of treatment, no energies are sent directly to another person. Moreover, as long as it's done properly, there is no infringement on the other person's free will.

Here's a suggested intent statement for a Reiki treatment directed at a failing or wounded relationship: "I ask that Reiki be sent to the relationship between myself and [insert name of other person here] to assist in mending our hearts and minds. This request is being made with the strongest intention that any healing that occurs will be for the highest good of all concerned."

Reiki Moon Rituals

The *Farmers' Almanac* warns that farmers should plant crops that produce their fruit above ground during the waxing moon. As for the crops that produce their fruit underground—like potatoes, carrots, turnips, and peanuts—they grow best when planted during the waning moon. Furthermore, the best time to harvest crops is during the waning moon, to ensure longer storage periods and freshest conditions.

The moon is said to be "waxing" as it proceeds from "new" to "first quarter" to "first gibbous" to "full" phase. The new-moon phase is the time when the face of the moon is completely in shadow. It is followed by the first-quarter phase, when the moon resembles a luminous half circle, its curved edge on the right side. The first-gibbous phase is when the moon appears as more than half-illuminated. The full phase is when the moon appears as a bright, luminous disk in the evening sky.

"Waning" of the moon occurs when it progresses from "full" to "last quarter" to "second gibbous" to "new" phase once again. The last-quarter phase occurs when the moon again appears as a half circle, but with its curved edge on the left side. The second-gibbous phase is when the moon again looks more than half-illuminated, as it does during the waxing period.

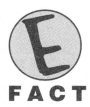

FACT

The sequence of moon phases repeats itself every 29 days, 12 hours, and 44 minutes. This cycle is known as the lunar month, or the synodic month.

Planting Our Ideas with Reiki

By looking to the moon phases as a guide for planting flowers and crops, we are ritualistically seeking the optimum harvest yields. Since we can employ the moon phases to figure out favorable time frames for sowing seeds, conceptually we can also use the moon cycles in planting our desires and ideas, as well as harvesting (manifesting) our goals and dreams.

Our intellectual seeds are planted during the new-moon phase. This is a time when our ideas and our desires begin to take form. As the new moon returns after the monthly lunar cycle, our ideas and desires begin to grow and eventually ripen. The full-moon phase is considered a time of completion and endings, when we get to harvest the outcomes of our labors and realize our dreams. It is also during the full moon that we can ritualistically release those aspects of ourselves that do not serve us well, such as addictions, greed, guilt, and fears.

Increasing and Decreasing Power

The Reiki Power symbol, Cho Ku Rei, is a complementary tool to use when participating in rituals scheduled according to the new and full phases of the moon. When the spiral action of the Cho Ku Rei is drawn counterclockwise, it increases power. When this action is reversed, and the Cho Ku Rei spiral is drawn clockwise, it decreases power. Increased Reiki power serves as the fertilizer that will nurture your personal seeds and seedlings, and also promotes the growth and maturity of your ideas. Decreased Reiki power can be used when we wish either to diminish or end those experiences and conditions in our lives that deplete our energies or overshadow our personal growth.

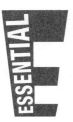

Wait until you have clarity before you call upon the universe to help you realize your dreams and desires. When your requests are ill-defined, the answers you had hoped for can be vague and the fulfillments just off the mark. Being nonspecific in your intention requests could result in unexpected and possibly even unpleasant surprises.

New-Moon Manifestation Ritual

New-moon manifestation ceremonies are implemented to expand the space within us and around us where our desires, wishes, good health, and well-being are created and realized. Before you embark upon this ritual, it is imperative that you know exactly what it is that you wish to manifest for yourself.

It is also recommended that your intention requests be stated as precisely as possible to ensure positive results. Any intention that is mentally focused on, voiced out loud, or written down on paper, carries power. That power is increased when the Cho Ku Rei symbol is visualized or drawn and either placed within or pressed upon that intention.

Here's what else you need to do to prepare for the Reiki new moon manifestation ritual:

- Check the calendar for the next upcoming new moon and schedule thirty minutes to perform the ritual.
- Gather your supplies. You will need a notebook, plastic transparency film, a colored pen or marker, and some cedar incense or a sage smudge wand.
- Prepare a clean and uncluttered sacred space, indoors or outdoors, where you will hold your new-moon ceremony.

Setting Your New-Moon Intentions in Motion

1. Cleanse your sacred area by saying an opening prayer honoring the Moon Mother. The Reiki Gassho prayer can also be incorporated at this time.
2. Clear away any lingering negative energies either with a sage smudging or by burning some cedar incense.
3. Imagine your right palm being dipped into a pan of colorful paint. Using that same hand, with your palm turned outward, paint the Cho Ku Rei symbol in the air at each corner of the room. If you are outdoors, paint the Power symbol in the air, directing it to the east, west, north, and south.
4. Center and ground your body by whatever means is most appropriate for you:
   a. Sit in quiet meditation.
   b. Light a lavender-scented candle.
   c. Drink a cup of chamomile or mint tea.
   d. Before or during the ceremony, intently ingest a blend of flower essences that offer grounding and manifesting properties.

5. Open your notebook and date it. Write down these (or similar) words: "I accept these things into my life now or something better for my highest good and for the highest good of all concerned." Below your intention statement, begin to write down a list of all your desires. Your list may consist of only one item or you may have several pages written down. Do not limit your list of items. Continually add other items to your list as often as you wish. If possessing many things in your life makes you happy and content, you should not deny yourself these things by limiting your requests.

6. With a marker, draw one or more Cho Ku Rei symbols on a sheet of plastic transparency film. Place the transparency film, with the Power symbols drawn upon it, on top of your hand-written list of requests. Close your notebook and put it away until next month's new moon, when you will reopen it and rededicate it.

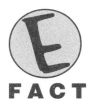

FACT

Some flower essences known to have manifestation properties are blackberry, cayenne, alfilaria, golden yarrow, hornbeam, Indian paintbrush, Shasta daisy, tansy, and walnut.

Changing Your New-Moon Intentions

Once you have laid out your new-moon intentions, do not feel that they have been set in stone. The moon has its phases and so do our personalities. Our needs and desires fluctuate depending on circumstance and life situations. Each month at the time of the new moon, rededicate your intention statement and your list of requests by repeating the Reiki new-moon manifestation ritual. Revise your list of intentions by rewriting the whole list on a fresh page of your notebook. Eliminate any items from your previous list that have come to fruition or no longer suit your needs or desires. You can also make any necessary changes to your list of intentions anytime before the moon has fully waxed. However, changes made midcycle will not have the benefit of the complete manifestation cycle.

Reiki Full-Moon Release Ceremony

The full moon represents completion. It indicates the end stage of any given period or cycle. During the time of the full moon, rituals are carried out to release or purge from our lives those things that do not serve us in a productive or useful manner. Such things might include addictions to food, drug abuse, or sexual dysfunction. By purging ourselves of these and other problems, we help relinquish sufferings associated with physical pains, emotional upsets, and hurtful relationships. Here's what you need to do in order to prepare for a Reiki full-moon release ritual:

- Check your calendar for the next upcoming full moon. Schedule a time, preferably in the evening after moonrise, to perform the full-moon release ceremony.
- Create a sacred space outdoors so that you will be illuminated by the moonlight during the ceremony.
- Gather your supplies. You'll need a fireproof cauldron, strips of writing paper, pen, clipboard, matches or candlelight, sage smudge wand, and water.

Setting Your Full-Moon Release in Motion

1. Cleanse your sacred area by reciting an opening prayer honoring the Moon Mother. The Reiki Gassho prayer can also be incorporated into the ceremony at this time.
2. Sit down and reflect on the things in your life that you wish to release or change. On separate slips of paper, write each item you wish to release or vow to change. (Use the clipboard for support.)
3. Read out loud what you have written on one strip of paper. Say these words (or something similar): "I release this now into the white light to be transformed into positive energies so that it can be used for universal good." Draw the Cho Ku Rei in reverse (clockwise) with your tongue on the roof of your mouth. Blow the tongue-drawn "decrease power symbol" onto the piece of paper. Light the paper using a match or candlelight and place it in a fireproof cauldron, where it will turn to ash.

4. Repeat step 3 for each strip of paper.
5. Cleanse your aura with the smoke from the sage wand. Thank the Earth Mother and your Reiki guides for the opportunity to release those things that no longer serve you. Use water to put out the smoldering ashes in the cauldron.

The Reiki Environment

In order to truly make Reiki a way of life, it is prudent to treat with Reiki all the environments in which you spend your time. Whether you are at home, work, the grocery market, health clinic, or anywhere else, you can increase the comfort level for yourself and everyone else in that environment simply by inviting Reiki to dwell there with you.

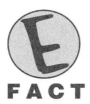

FACT

Giving Reiki to any designated space is an interesting experiment for you to try. Results will vary, depending on the current energy state of the particular space you select and of the occupants of that space. Optionally, you can send Reiki in advance to any place you plan to visit later by visualizing the symbols and directing a distant treatment.

Home Sweet Home

Your primary goal may be to make your own home a Reiki haven. Basically, you can infuse your home with Reiki healing energies by touching everything in sight. Reiki your house plants, family pets, the furniture, and appliances. Reiki the entryways, stairwells, closets, and pantries. Reiki the bed pillows and mattresses. The list of tangibles that you can infuse with the energy of Reiki within your home is endless.

Reiki Anywhere and Everywhere

As previously discussed, Reiki will turn on automatically whenever and wherever it is needed. Reiki will flow out from a practitioner to another person who is receptive to its energies whenever these two are in the same environment. If you know in advance that you are going to be at a certain place, send distant Reiki to that place beforehand in order to help create a more receptive and healing environment for you to visit. Before visiting a home, school, store, or office building, employ the absentia formula to send Reiki to those places.

Before walking into any sort of building, visualize a large Reiki Power symbol drawn in the building's entrance doorway. As you enter the building, you will walk through this freshly drawn Power symbol. Walking through eight-foot-tall Cho Ku Rei symbols can feel extremely empowering.

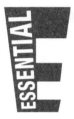

When traveling, you can incorporate the use of Reiki's Protection symbol as a cautionary measure to help safeguard your luggage and its contents from loss or damage.

Planes, Trains, and Automobiles

Traveling can be a tedious, stressful experience filled with anxiety and tension. Travelers face a variety of conditions that can prove upsetting. Among these are traffic jams, canceled flights, missed connections, lost baggage, and many other aggravations. Panicky emotions associated with these types of mishaps—as well as bouts of motion sickness—can wreak havoc on our nervous systems.

Reiki is an excellent tool for keeping our traveling stresses to a minimum. Self-treatments as well as distant treatments are wonderfully relaxing and healing for passengers traveling in airplanes, trains, buses, and automobiles. The travel-weary Reiki practitioner knows that whenever he or she is on the road and traveling for extended periods of time, there is a comfortable hotel with a bed to crash in at the end of each long day of travel. And where there is a bed, there is a full-body Reiki treatment waiting to happen. Happy trails!

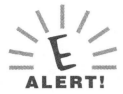
ALERT!

It is not recommended that you send distant Reiki to anyone who may be driving a car or operating heavy machinery. The relaxing nature of Reiki is known to cause drowsiness, which could cause an accident. The driver needs to be as wide-awake as possible in order to focus his or her full attention on operating the motor vehicle.

Past, Present, and Future Events

Living in the moment is a challenge we are all faced with. Although most of us don't realize it, we seldom live our lives in the present. At various times throughout any given day, our thoughts tend to drift back and forth from our past experiences to our future planned events. While we are mentally revisiting childhood memories or needlessly fretting about next week's deadline at work, we overlook the "here and now" of our life today.

Reiki has access to both your past and your future. It will flow beyond present-day ailments, delving deeply into the body to heal past hurts. And Reiki's distant formula can also be used to offer positive energies to future events.

In the Past

It is our past experiences that have helped form our personalities. Who we are today, or, put another way, what we have made of ourselves, is the result of the culmination of all our past experiences. Reiki can be directed at specific memories to heal energies surrounding those experiences that negatively influence the current personality.

The Reiki Connection symbol, Hon Sha Ze Sho Nen, gives the adept Reiki practitioner the tool to assist him or her in accessing the Akashic Records. Here the practitioner can obtain information on hurts and ills that are lingering in the body from past experiences. These lingering hurts may date back to last week, last month, last year, or much farther back in time—as far back as your childhood and past-life experiences.

For example, Reiki can be directed to treat the lingering fear of a person who had a traumatic first day at school. This is an example of "inner-child therapy." You can use a teddy bear surrogate to facilitate your own inner-child work. Rather than doing a full-body treatment, sit quietly with a stuffed teddy bear on your lap or hold a hand-sized bear between the palms of your hands. Use the distant formula and send Reiki to the small child within you that needs love, understanding, and healing. Spend at least a full hour on this to fully give your inner child the care that he or she desperately craves.

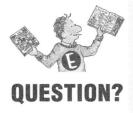

QUESTION?

What are the Akashic Records?
The Akashic Records, also known as The Book of Life, may be described as the vibrational volumes where every experience (thought, action, and emotion) of every soul in existence is recorded. It is the database that psychics explore to glean prophetic and past-life information.

In the Future

The distant treatment formula takes a forward leap when Reiki is utilized to energize future events. Sending Reiki ahead to smooth the way for you before embarking on a particular venture or journeying to a specific place is an excellent confidence builder. Here are a few examples of future events that you may wish to energize using Reiki distant treatment:

- Academic exams
- Blind dates
- Family gatherings
- Giving birth
- Job interviews
- Medical appointments
- School reunions
- Speaking engagements
- Sports tournaments
- Talent shows

You won't feel as lonely, fearful, or lost if confronted with new experiences when you have Reiki energies awaiting you to make your transition into a strange or uncomfortable situation easier. The Reiki warms up the space and helps your communications with others as future events unfold.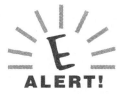

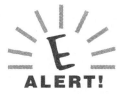

Reiki is limited only by our limited actions in using it. It will support us while we grudgingly perform our daily chores. Reiki will also energize us when we are pursuing our hobbies and playing with our friends.

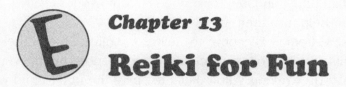

Chapter 13

Reiki for Fun

The routines of daily life can become a chore when we don't take time out for play and when we take everything too seriously. If you read the comics before you read the front-page news, or if you prefer to enjoy your dessert before you eat the main course, you will enjoy the joyous and spirit-loving ways in which Reiki can be integrated into your hobbies and playtime. Reiki's love energies can lift your spirits, tantalize your palate, spice up your sex life, and help make your dreams come true.

In Your Reiki Sandbox

A sandbox is a positive image—it's a fun place where children's creative abilities are sparked. Or it may be a less-positive image—a giant kitty litter box for the homeless felines in your neighborhood. It all depends on what perspective you choose to take. Do you view half a glass of water as half empty or half full? Imposing Reiki energies onto your negative perspectives can help turn them into positives.

Children are extremely receptive to Reiki's energies. One of the reasons why this is true is because children spend more hours every day playing than they do working. Allow Reiki to spark the inner child within you and it will bring more joy and happiness into your life. All work and no play makes for a very dreary existence, and it can drag you down emotionally. With Reiki as your companion, you will soon be building towering sandcastles as high as the skies.

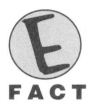

FACT

Reiki flows spontaneously whenever we work creatively with our hands—when we are gardening, landscaping, playing musical instruments, painting, writing, sewing, quilting, sculpting, or carving wood.

Better Than a Green Thumb

Universal Life Energy courses through all forms of living things—plants, animals, fungi, protists, and even bacteria and viruses. Whether you are a learned horticulturist, a greenhouse enthusiast, a window box gardener, or merely someone who enjoys nurturing a couple of small houseplants, complementing your gardening talents with Reiki energies will color your thumb a shade or two greener.

Plants will thrive when they've got sufficient supplies of sunshine and water—and even more so if you feed them with Reiki. Reiki will naturally flow through your palms whenever you are handling seeds and plants. You may also place Reiki energies in water and organic fertilizers before administering nourishment to your plants. This can be done by either immersing your hands directly into the water or by grasping the watering pitcher in both your hands to allow Reiki to penetrate through the container.

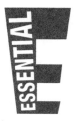

Surprise your favorite gardener by giving him or her a plant or botanical gift basket filled with goodies that have been charged with Reiki. Place Reiki energies and the Reiki symbols over all the gift items: potted plant, seed packets, garden gloves, clay flowerpot, and potting soil.

Reiki a Tree

You've heard the phrase "hug a tree" before, but have you ever taken a moment to actually do this? All trees need a hug now and again. Trees are also extremely receptive to Reiki energies and will soak up tremendous amounts when it is applied. As Reiki flows through your body into the intricate root system and expansive, towering branches of a tree, the experience will be both grounding and uplifting. Here is how you can find the perfect tree to hug and bestow with Reiki:

- Find a quiet park, forest, or woodland area.
- Walk among the trees until you feel comfortable in their presence.
- Feel the different bark textures with the palms of your hands.
- Smell the scent of the various woods.
- Absorb the earth's ki energies as you stand among the trees and look upward to their sprawling branches overhead.
- Find the perfect tree that fits your mood. You will know which one is right for you when you feel the warmth and resurgence of Reiki energies swelling up in your palms.

You can share several types of hugs:

1. **Vertical tree hug:** Encircle the tree with your arms while gently pressing your cheek to the trunk, being careful not to scratch your face. Squeeze tightly. Sigh deeply. Place your palms firmly upon the tree bark. Reiki your tree.

2. **Full-body tree hug:** Sit on the ground, wrapping your legs around the base of the tree and at the same time embracing it with your arms. Place your palms firmly upon the tree bark. Reiki your tree.

3. **Up-in-the-air tree hug:** Climb a tree. Sit upon a strong limb and straddle it. Bend forward and place your belly against it while wrapping your arms about it. Place your palms firmly upon the tree bark. Reiki your tree.

When you give Reiki to a tree, you will notice how your tree magnificently returns the favor by sending regenerated Reiki energies back to you. Be one with your tree.

Reiki the Earth's Natural Resources

Ki is the life-breath of all living creatures and their ecosystems here on earth. Any time you offer Reiki energy to the earth's natural resources, it will be openly and graciously accepted. Offer Reiki to the forests, oceans, prairies, mountains, hillsides, rivers, lakes and ponds, deserts, farmlands, and orchards. It will make you feel less isolated and help you to better understand your connection to every living thing.

Diet and Nutrition

Body image and overall dietary health concerns are prominent in today's society. Like all eclectic groups of people, Reiki practitioners come in all shapes and sizes—heavyset and thin, tall and short, and in all varying degrees and combinations of body types.

Because of Reiki's balancing properties, it is not surprising that some practitioners have experimented using Reiki as a determining factor in making their nutritional decisions. Here are a couple of different ways you can place Reiki's Power symbols in your meals to empower your dietary intake:

1. **Increase power:** Visualize or draw the Power symbol, a counter-clockwise spiral, in the air. Place the symbol in your food before

eating your meals with the intention to *increase* the energetic volume of the food. Each bite you eat will be more filling and you will be satisfied with eating smaller portions.

2. **Decrease power:** Visualize or draw the reverse Power symbol, a clockwise spiral, in the air. Place the symbol in your food before eating your meals with the intention to *decrease* your appetite. Your meals will no longer be as appealing to you and you will invariably eat less.

It is a good habit to bless and vitalize your food with Reiki. The blessing action is meant to serve as a Reiki treatment that will discharge any harmful toxins or impurities from the food before it is consumed. To Reiki your food, simply place your hands over the dinner plate for a few seconds before you begin eating. Foods that are in serving dishes meant for the whole family can be blessed with Reiki before they are passed around the dinner table. If you are the person who prepares and cooks the meals for your family, you can also Reiki the food during the preparation and cooking process.

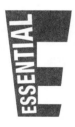

If you wish to discreetly offer Reiki blessings to your meals when you are in a public place or restaurant, simply place your hands, palms up, on your lap under the table. The Reiki energies will flow upward through the tabletop and through the dinner plate in order to reach your food.

Food Testing

Some people are trained in using muscle testing for identifying allergies and sensitivities to foods. Similarly, Reiki can be used in determining which foods are good or bad for you. Reiki tests can be conducted once you become adept in reading the varying temperatures and velocities of Reiki's energies.

Scan your palm over a particular food and allow Reiki to evaluate it for you. For some practitioners, hot and faster-flowing energy from the palm indicates a good food choice for them. In contrast, a cooler and slower flow would indicate a poor food choice. For others, the cooler and slower flow indicates a positive reading, and the warmer and faster flow is a negative reading. With practice, each person will be able to determine what type of response indicates a positive or negative reading for him or her.

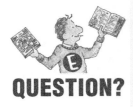

QUESTION?

What is muscle testing?
Sometimes referred to as applied kinesiology, muscle testing is an evaluation system that involves reading responses from a muscular tissue of the body when slight pressure is applied to it. Self-testing can be done to obtain information on many subjects, including the diagnosis of nutritional deficiencies and food sensitivities.

Calories and Calisthenics

Reducing calories in your daily diet and increasing the amount of exercise you do is the surest way to lose weight. Vitalizing your meals with Reiki will not reduce the number of calories in foods before you eat them. However, when we Reiki our meals, we raise the vibrational levels of these foods. The life force within us is increased when we ingest foods that have been vitalized with Reiki. As a result, these foods will be more easily digested, providing increased energy to the body. When we feel energized, we are more inclined to make exercise become a routine.

Food Indulgences

Most of us find that there can be much pleasure derived from eating our favorite foods. There is certainly nothing wrong with nourishing our bodies and satisfying our taste buds with foods we enjoy, as long as overindulging does not become the end result. There is a wide difference between nourishing our bodies and abusing them by stuffing them with excess and empty calories. If you are in a treatment program for an eating disorder or food addiction, Reiki will complement that treatment by assisting you in overcoming the problem as well as in helping you make the correct dietary choices.

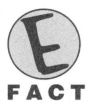

FACT

Following mealtimes, Reiki hands placed on the solar plexus for three to five minutes will stimulate the digestive process within the body to function more effectively. It is also important to drink plenty of water to flush the toxins from the body. Be sure to Reiki your drinking water.

Let Reiki Be Your Shopping Guru

People will often take a friend along with them on their shopping excursions in order to have a second opinion before purchasing items. We don't always trust our own judgments in knowing what color or style of clothing best suits us. Unfortunately, Reiki is not the fashion guru of the century. However, you can rely on Reiki to clue you in on which melon is the freshest at the market or which flowering shrub at the garden center will grow the best in your soil.

Once you've learned to read its language, you will never again go shopping without using Reiki as your shopping guide. Basically, you can scan any living thing that has ki energies running through it to get a positive or negative reading on it. Living things that can be scanned before you purchase them include foods, natural drinks, herbs, essential oils, flower essences, vitamins, medications, crystals and gemstones, plants, and even pets.

Mood Enhancement and Meditation

Mind-body connection studies have proved that a regular course of meditation improves the function of the immune system as well as offering other medical benefits. Meditation techniques may include any of the following:

- Vocalizing repetitive mantras
- Listening to music

- Practicing imagery and visualization
- Participating in active meditative-style exercises such as dance, Kundalini yoga, and tai chi

Reiki energies complement all meditative approaches that people use to promote well-being.

Reiki Visualization Vacation

Whether you need to quash depressive thoughts or calm overstimulated nerves, imaginative visualization may be the solution. If you find it easy to mentally visualize the Reiki symbols, you will enjoy playing with these symbols during your meditations. Imagery play can be a welcome escape from the mundane or frustrating events and toils of daily life. Although it is not advisable to have your head in the clouds or buried in the sand on a regular basis, taking short visual vacations away from your stressful life can certainly revive depressive moods.

Take a ten-minute break from reality and let your imagination carry you away to a trouble-free space. Allow the Reiki Connection symbol, Hon Sha Ze Sho Nen, to be the "magic carpet" that carries you off to faraway places. Focus on a desired destination, draw the symbol, and mentally send the energy to that place, with yourself tagging along for the ride.

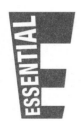

Pamper yourself with a Reiki bath. Before stepping into the tub for a relaxing soak, enhance your bathing experience by charging your bath water and all your bath supplies with Reiki. Bath products you can charge with Reiki include sponges, loofas, bubble bath gel, soap, and bath salts.

Another imaginative visualization you can try is to imagine a large Hula-Hoop floating horizontally in the air above you. The hoop represents a vortex opening into a different reality. Visualize the Power symbol, Cho Ku Rei, floating inside the circular hoop. Next, imagine yourself jumping up into the hoop and through the Power symbol into a new reality of your making. This reality can be a revisitation to your childhood, a swim date with a school of dolphins, or an explorative tour through an enchanted castle. With the help of this visualization, you can go virtually anywhere your mind will take you.

Pumping Ki

Breath awareness exercises and physical workouts are two excellent activities that will help open up your ki passages prior to giving or receiving a Reiki treatment. Choose exercises that remind you of play—most people tend to prefer activities that are joyous and fun to those that feel laborious or bothersome.

A favorite ki breath exercise is to open your mouth, relax your jaw, stick out your tongue, and pant like a dog. The in-and-out breaths will open up your belly and clear the ki passageways from the base of your spine to your throat's vocal cords.

An enjoyable physical exercise that will free up knots and kinks in the spine is to rock your body back and forth like a rocking chair. Position your body comfortably on a yoga mat or carpeted floor. Bend your knees and bring them close to your chest. Wrap your arms around your knees and begin rocking your body back and forth. This movement massages your back's bones and muscles. It also effectively opens up the ki channels that run along your spine. Best of all, it's easy and simply fun to do, almost like being a kid again!

Book a Reiki Session

Doing self-treatments is a wonderful way to value yourself and to honor your body, but sometimes we crave touch and caring from another individual in order to feel fully loved and pampered. Swapping treatments with other practitioners is one option. If you are traveling or visiting a new town, try to locate a Reiki practitioner in the area and treat yourself to a full-body treatment. You may discover a new friend as well as learn a new healing technique in the process. It will also make your stay in a strange place more pleasurable.

Reiki and Your Sex Life

One of the myths instilled in some spiritual teachings is that the physical body is a hindrance to our spiritual development. We already *are* spiritual beings, first and foremost. Our physical bodies allow us, as spiritual beings, to experience human existence. Why would we strive to shed our physical garb and lose the opportunity to have this unique experience?

Choosing celibacy over sexuality will not make a person more spiritual than a person who enjoys sexual intimacy. Celibacy is a choice, but it is only one pathway a person can choose to take in experiencing life. As a choice, celibacy does have some merits. It offers an experience that can help a person develop his or her personal awareness. Those who choose celibacy feel that their choice is more "spiritually appropriate" for them, but it's not a superior choice. Some Reiki practitioners choose celibacy, while others are sexually active. Neither group is more superior or more spiritual than the other.

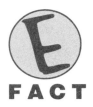

FACT

The sacral chakra determines our sexual appetites and disposition. It is also associated with our playfulness and our creative natures. Spiritual lessons associated with the sacral chakra are creativity, manifestation, honoring relationships, and learning to "let go."

Ruled by the Sacral Chakra

The attunement process that activates Reiki moves the ki energies through all the chakras. The energy movement begins at the crown chakra and moves downward through the root chakra and back up again. Any chakras that are shut down or partially blocked will be opened up during the attunement. The second chakra, the body's sexual center, cannot help but be affected by this. This is especially true if it has not been functioning fully beforehand. If a person has been sexually repressed or has had his sexual center shut down, the Reiki attunement could very possibly open up a "Pandora's box" of intimacy-related issues, sexual urges, and emotions.

A person can have an active sex life even when his sacral chakra is blocked or shut down. Basically, a person with a closed sexual center goes through the motion of having sex without having a total awareness of his body. Having sex in this way can be enjoyable, but it does not compare to having a sexual experience with the sacral chakra open. Sharing sexual intimacy while your sacral chakra is open and functioning can be a completely startling experience for someone who has been closed off from his or her physical body. Admittedly, being fully in your body while making love can be exhilarating, to say the least. You will not likely forget the feeling once you have experienced it because it is a glorious blend of the physical and the spiritual.

Turning Your Partner On with Reiki

Reiki and sexual intimacy go together beautifully. The Reiki practitioner who conducts regular self-treatments will keep his or her chakras spinning and purring in perfect working order. When your sacral chakra is open and functioning, it can work like an "attraction beacon" that will bring together you and your lover like a pair of magnets. Your lover may not realize why she is being drawn so strongly to you; she will just know that being around you makes her feel good.

Bringing Reiki energy into your lovemaking is not only a wonderful gift for yourself but will also be appreciated by your partner. If, by chance, you and your partner are both attuned to Reiki, your lovemaking has the potential to blend your energies together in sacred sexuality; in other words, it will be a union of two souls.

Reiki Body Massage

Giving your partner a Reiki massage is an openhearted and nurturing demonstration of your love. For some couples, it may be a good way to arouse each other sexually. For others, it may have a calming, relaxing effect, easing the stresses from the recipient's body and sending them right into a slumber pose. Whether you use it for foreplay or *foresleep,* Reiki massage is a wonderful way to be intimate with your partner.

The basic Reiki hand placements are not used while giving a

massage. Reiki will naturally kick in during the session. For instance, you can lovingly give your partner a Reiki back rub:

1. Charge your (preferably organic) massage oils with Reiki energies. Sweet almond oil and jojoba oil are favorites for releasing stresses.
2. Have your partner lay on her stomach on the bed.
3. Cover the lower part of your partner's body with some warm towels so she will not be chilled.
4. Pour a handful of massage oil in your hands. Allow your Reiki hands to warm the oil.
5. Begin by smoothing your hands in slow, sweeping movements across your partner's neck, shoulders, and upper back.
6. Begin stroking and rubbing the neck and shoulders.
7. Continue kneading out any kinks or stresses as you move your hands down your partner's back.
8. Finish the massage by lightly scratching her skin surface with your fingernails in circular or figure-eight movements.
9. Lie down and snuggle up next to your partner.

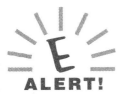

ALERT!

The back rub massage described here should not be used as therapy in a clinical setting or as a healing practice. Such behavior is not acceptable between a practitioner and a client and should be reserved for your intimate relationship.

Enjoying Life with Reiki

Allowing Reiki energies to be woven into your creative hobbies and playtime is simply another way to understand the flexibility of this healing art. Reiki is not merely a healing practice that demands inflexible rules or strict values. On the contrary, it is an art of fluidity that offers a variety of different expressions to the many people who use it.

Reiki will adapt to your needs no matter whether they are serious or lighthearted. Are you documenting your Reiki achievements, manifestations, and success stories? If not, the next chapter will help you get started.

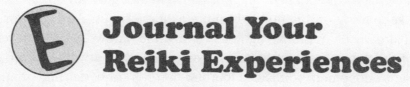

Chapter 14

Journal Your Reiki Experiences

For centuries, people have been relying on diaries, travelogues, and scrapbooks to document their histories, pilgrimages, experiences, and individual insights. Recording your Reiki experiences by writing them down in a notebook or private journal is a good way to track energy shifts and personal growth changes that occur. Your Reiki journal need not be anything fancy, nor need your scribblings be profound. Simply jot down notes in a handy pocket notebook, keep a private diary, or publish an online blog.

Dedicating Your Journal

For every adventure embarked upon there is both anticipation and apprehension surrounding it. You may experience ambiguous emotions because you're not sure how and why events and experiences will eventually unfold. Being newly attuned to Reiki is very much like starting a "new page" or "chapter" in your life. Why not grab an empty notebook and keep a log of this new adventure as it plays out? And for those who have already been practicing Reiki for a while, know that it is never too late to pick up the habit of keeping a journal. Even if you have not yet begun to document your Reiki journey, there is no better time than now.

Materials Needed

At the start of any new endeavor, it is meaningful to make some advance preparations. Have some fun gathering the supplies you will need to keep a creative journal. Do you remember the excitement you felt when shopping for the required school supplies at the start of a new school year? With a new supply of loose-leaf paper, notebooks, pens, pencils, and ruler in hand, you welcomed the opportunity for a "fresh start" in the next grade.

To help you keep your journal, you may need the following supplies:

- Notebook or sketchpad
- Loose-leaf paper and a three-ring binder
- Paper hole-puncher
- Colored markers or highlighters
- Glue or rubber cement
- Scissors and ruler
- Pens and pencils
- Sheet protectors
- Index cards

Choosing a notebook with unruled paper will give you the flexibility to be creative. Blank books are readily available in bookstores, art supply stores, and department stores. If you prefer to type out some of your journal entries using a word-processing program, you will need a hole puncher and three-ring binder with page dividers to organize your printed computer pages.

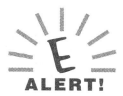

ALERT!

You are a work in process, or, in other words, you are growing with Reiki. The journal will serve as a yardstick that measures how tall you've grown and will continue to grow.

How to Begin—Step One

After selecting a notebook, binder, or journal book to use for your Reiki writings, your first step is to put your own unique identifying mark on it. Fill the first couple of pages with information about yourself and what your reasons are for bringing Reiki into your life. Paste a photograph of yourself on the cover or on the inside cover of the journal. This journal is about Reiki, but more so, its purpose is to track your Reiki pilgrimage. The primary focus of keeping a Reiki journal is *you* and your personal experiences and sentiments when using Reiki. You and Reiki are the two staple ingredients in this endeavor, with you serving as the storyteller. It is important that you recognize your own value in this process.

How to Begin—Step Two

After you personalize your journal, the second step is for you to write down your reasons for taking a Reiki class and what your initial expectations are for choosing Reiki. Write down your impressions of your teacher. What types of emotions were you feeling during the class? Describe your reactions to the attunement process. Did you sense a rapport with any of your classmates, or did you sense agitations with some classmates?

Continue to write, write, and write some more. Don't worry if you are rambling or wandering off subject. You are not writing a manuscript that is going to be published. This journal-keeping exercise is meant for your own personal use. Think of it as a private forum where you can express your feelings freely. No one is going to grade it or reprove you for messy handwriting.

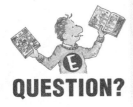

What is a blog?
A blog is a journal that is created using a special computer software program. The program allows a user to make daily journal entries that are instantaneously published on the Internet for either public or private (password-protected) viewing.

How to Begin—Step Three

The third step is to write out an intention statement. Make your intention statement as clear and concise as possible to ensure it can't be misunderstood. Here are a few sample intention statements, although you should certainly feel free to make up your own:

- It is my intent to use Reiki in my life in order to develop a deeper relationship with my personal awareness.
- I choose to embrace Reiki with all that I am.
- It is my intent to create a healthier, wealthier, and happier life for me and my family.

Follow your intention statement with a brief dedication. Here are a few sample suggestions:

- I dedicate this book to my Reiki guides and the inner child within me who wants to get out and play more often.
- I dedicate this book to my Reiki Master and my own journey following her wise and wandering footsteps.
- This Reiki journal is dedicated to the creativity that stirs within me. May I always pursue joy.

Bless your Reiki journal by holding it between both your hands and allowing Reiki energies to flow freely from your palms into its pages. If you've been attuned to Level II Reiki, you may also add Reiki symbols in your journal. Keep your book in a handy place, such as inside your desk drawer or on top of your bedside table, where you can readily find it and add entries to it on a regular basis.

Letting Creativity Flow

You have completed steps one, two, and three. Now the instruction ends. There are no steps numbered four, five, and six. The continuation of this journal project is entirely up to you. Actually, you can ignore steps one, two, and three, if you like, and create your own steps to begin with. Those initial three steps are only meant as a framework to get you started.

The true treasure within creative journal writing is that there are no steadfast rules. A poet will fill his journal with impromptu prose and beautiful poetry. The artist's journal pages will be adorned with drawings and sketches. The neat pin will likely keep her journal tidy and well organized, with little fluff or doodle clutter. The free-spirited individual will sprinkle his notebook with frills and spontaneous journal entries. Your goals should be to express your emotions and to document your Reiki experiences.

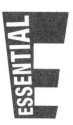

Your journal doesn't have to be filled with pages and pages of text. You can add drawings, doodles, and diagrams if that will help you better express yourself. Keep a set of markers or colored pencils next to your journal, and use them to enhance your written entries whenever the mood strikes you.

Ready, Set, Go!

After you have dedicated your journal and have begun to fill up its pages, it is entirely up to you what types of entries you wish to include in your journal. Document your self-treatments by sharing your treatment intentions and the sensations experienced as a result of each session. Use your journal as a sketchpad to draw the Reiki symbols or draw the things you wish to make a reality in your life. Record Reiki requests that you receive from your friends and family members. Describe your challenges, frustrations, and confusions. Also journal your successes, fulfilled dreams, and lessons learned. Continue to write out new and modified scripts of "intention statements" as your personal needs and desires change.

Scissors and Glue

Get crazy! Engage in some scrapbooking techniques to enhance your journal with some sparkle and color. Expand your handwritten journal by pasting in cutouts that visually represent those things that you hope to make a reality in your life. After all, a picture can convey as clear a message as any written intention. When you see an image in a catalog or newspaper that depicts something that you would like to have, clip it out and paste it into your book. For example, if you wish to take a romantic Alaskan cruise, paste a picture of a cruise ship alongside another picture of an igloo and the ocean. Write the words "Alaskan cruise for two" between these two images in order to complete your focused intention.

Personal Growth

Our expectations and perspectives change as our lives advance. This is true whether or not you make Reiki a part of your life. However, with Reiki's involvement these changes often progress more quickly. In many cases the regular application of Reiki treatments quickens personal growth. Changes that would ordinarily take a long time to come to fruition will be hastened to completion, so that you're able to secure a healthier and more empowering life sooner rather than later or not at all.

It can be remarkably interesting to turn the pages back to your first journal entries a few weeks, months, or perhaps years after they were written and review your recorded thoughts and feelings about your Reiki experiences. Sometimes we are impatient, feeling as if we are spinning our wheels in this life. We want changes to occur instantly. Going back in time and reading your early journal entries will help you better understand that life has not stood still. The concerns and troubles that were bothering you early on will likely not seem so important or overwhelming to you later. In fact, many of those ruts in the road and tricky stumbling blocks will have faded away completely. You will discover that your goals and initiatives will have been met or ultimately changed to something entirely different. Our priorities change as life advances. Reiki can help put all of our priorities in order.

The Postattunement Journal

Following the attunement ceremony, a Reiki practitioner goes through a purification period for a number of days. Traditionally, this period of time is said to last for twenty-one days. Changes that occur during this period can be quite noticeable (see Chapter 4). Some Reiki teachers suggest to their students that they keep a journal or chart to document these changes. Common changes are adjustments in diet and sleep such as a desire to fast, cravings for certain types of food, insomnia, or sleepiness.

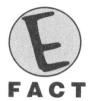

FACT

The twenty-one-day purification period is symbolic of the number of days that Dr. Mikao Usui, the founder of Reiki, held his meditation fast on Mt. Kurama. It was on the twenty-first day on the mountain that he rediscovered Reiki.

Following is a template for a chart that you can use to track your purification period. Use a ruler and pencil to draft the chart on one or two pages of your journal. Another option is to set up a spreadsheet program on your computer. When the twenty-one-day period is over, print it out, punch holes in the paper, and insert it into your three-ring binder.

The chart would continue on to day 21. After you go through the detoxification process, you will be able to look back on what you've experienced and how your body dealt with being attuned.

Documenting Reiki Sessions

Tracking your Reiki self-treatments by recording or documenting them is advantageous to your continued practice of Reiki. By reviewing your notes, you will get concrete clues as to what healing techniques work best for you. You may also learn what time of the day is more favorable for conducting treatments, better understand what kinds of results can be realized, and begin to carve out basic groundwork that will benefit future treatments.

Your Reiki journal is certainly a good place to record your self-treatment observations. Treatment notations can be blended into your

Sample Twenty-One-Day Purification Journal

Day Countdown	Reiki Self-Treatment	Hours of Sleep	Food Intake	Notes
Day 1	yes	9	orange juice, tomato soup, cheese wafers, strawberry milk shake	4 attunements for Reiki Level I; feelings of joy; sleepiness
Day 2	yes	5	toast with peanut butter, tuna fish on whole wheat, sliced peaches, veggie burger, fried potato wedges with onions	feeling full of energy
Day 3	yes	4	onion bagel with cream cheese, applesauce, carrot sticks, pork loin, vegetable medley	feeling full of energy; insomnia
Day 4	yes	8	oatmeal, orange juice, chef salad, French onion soup, garlic toast, chocolate cake	crying jag; emotional release
Day 5	no	10	corn flakes, skim milk, turkey sub, lentil soup	low energy; telephoned mother; 2-hour afternoon nap
Day 6	no	8½	orange juice, bran muffin, peanut butter and jelly sandwich, fish filet, creamed corn, butterscotch pudding	constipation; craving sweets
Day 7	yes	7½	oatmeal, orange juice, melon, grapes, wheat crackers, chicken and broccoli casserole, pear half	energetic; vivid dream about brightly colored kites flying in the sunny sky

other journal entries. Label or highlight them in some way so that they can easily be identified as you thumb through your journal pages. If you are using a three-ring binder, you may find it helpful to keep a separate divider section for your self-treatment notes.

Some practitioners prefer not to use a book journal when recording their Reiki treatment notes. Here are some different ideas for keeping your treatment notations:

- **Index cards**—Use one index card to record information about each treatment. You can file the cards by date or by intention.
- **Tape recording**—Following each treatment, make an audio recording of yourself discussing the treatment's details. This method is a good option for anyone who has difficulty expressing his or her feelings on paper.
- **Spreadsheets**—You can take advantage of your computer to chart your Reiki treatments. Spreadsheet columns can be labeled with "Date of Treatment," "My Intention Statement," "Sensations," "My Notes," and "Treatment Results."

As you begin to give Reiki treatments to others, you can use these same techniques to preserve your observations or sensations that may occur during your sessions.

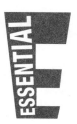

You can send a handwritten Reiki love letter to your significant other. Simply charge the paper and pen with Reiki energies before you write down your sentiments. Hold your completed love letter between the palms of your hands to infuse it with more Reiki love energies before sending it off to your partner.

Recording Reiki Requests

Aside from maintaining a personal Reiki journal, you may also want to keep an additional notebook for recording any Reiki requests that come your way. Basically the contents of this notebook will consist of a laundry list of names and requests. Each time someone asks you to send them absentia Reiki treatments, jot down the person's name along with the specific request that was given inside your Reiki request notebook.

When you do your distant treatments, open your book and read the new entries. Using the distant formula, send Reiki energies with the intention that the energies be dispersed to each individual listed in your notebook. Reiki will then go out to everyone listed, including new entries as well as those whose names were added in earlier entries. Older entries can be crossed out when they are no longer applicable.

Optionally, you can write out the Reiki requests on individual slips of paper. Afterward, you can tack the individual requests onto a bulletin board or place them inside a ceramic pot or wooden box. When sending distant Reiki energies, you will direct them to the bulletin board, ceramic pot, or wooden box. From time to time you can clear away older requests that are no longer relevant. You can read more about distant Reiki treatments in Chapter 8.

Dreams and Manifestations

Think of your journal as the perfect garden spot wherein you lovingly nurture and elegantly cultivate your expressed dreams and desires. Reiki is one of the grandest manifestation tools available today and can be very powerful. Reiki manifestations will even work for those "seeing is believing" types if they are willing to give it a try. All you need to do is follow these simple steps:

1. Dream it.
2. Write it down.
3. Stamp your intention on it.
4. Focus on it.
5. Apply Reiki to it.
6. It manifests!

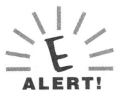

Naturally, Reiki manifestations can be limited or blocked. But they are only limited or blocked because of the limits or barriers that we impose on them. Those limitations and barriers are of our own making and never originate within Reiki itself.

Focusing on the Positives

When written down, our dreams and wants will thrive and soak up Reiki energies within our journal pages. We are planting the seeds of intent. We are pronouncing to the universe what will make us happiest.

Often, the things that we focus on are actualized in our lives. What is troubling is that we often focus on the things that make us unhappy. Even if you know this to be true, breaking the habit of focusing on negatives isn't always so easy.

Because of Reiki's "no harm" energies, it does not support the negatives that we may focus on. Reiki will not feed negative thoughts. This is a good thing and reason alone to have Reiki as your constant daily companion.

Reiki Affirmations

Sprinkle your journal with handwritten affirmations. When writing your own affirmations, make sure that you keep the sentence structure in present tense. Don't use words or phrases that imply a future time, such as "I will," "I wish," or "I want." Instead, pick phrases that imply the present, such as "I am," "I do," or "I choose." Feel free to use any of the affirmations listed here for your own personal Reiki journal:

- I am love.
- I am power.
- I am wealthy.
- I am wise.
- Peace radiates from inside me and all around me.
- I allow the power of love to enrich my life.
- I send all negativity away to be carried off in a bubble. I allow this bubble to return to me after all negative thoughts have been transmuted into positive energy.
- Creating an abundant life is my birthright. In this moment and from now on I claim my birthright.
- I am an active participant in my own mental health and well-being.

- My success is limitless.
- I choose my words carefully to create positive experiences for myself and for all those with whom I share my life. My words are powerful and loving!
- In my own special way I contribute to the world and make it a better place.
- I play an important role in the universe.
- Love abounds because of my daily efforts. I rejoice in doing ordinary tasks. I am beyond ordinary. I am unique.
- I live my dreams.

Your Recorded History

Our histories are passed down to new generations through documented facts and stories. When our experiences are not recorded, our memories tend to blur. When undocumented accounts of stories are retold weeks, months, or years later, our memories are often unreliable and inaccuracies in the storytelling occur.

Keep your Reiki memories accurate by writing down your stories while they are still fresh in your mind. Through these stories, you will be able to share the many benefits of Reiki with generations to come. Ⓔ

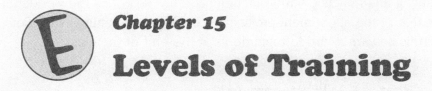

Chapter 15

Levels of Training

There are three levels of basic training in Usui Reiki: Level I, Level II, and Level III. At the highest level, you may become a Master/Teacher, but being certified in the highest level does not necessarily reflect superior knowledge. It is through the continued practice of Reiki that one becomes proficient. The Level I practitioner who uses Reiki daily will be more aware of how Reiki works than a Level III Reiki Master/Teacher who seldom conducts treatments.

Getting Certified

The Reiki student is attuned to Reiki during his or her classroom session through an initiation ceremony that is traditionally passed down from Master/Teacher to student. The attunement process is what makes Reiki stand apart from other types of healing-touch systems. Although other healing arts may use hand placements, only Reiki has the wonderful benefit of the attunement process. At each level of attunement, Reiki certificates are awarded to students at the end of the class.

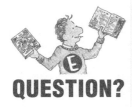

QUESTION?

What is a Reiki attunement?
A Reiki attunement is a ritual that is performed by the Reiki Master/Teacher. Through a specific set of sequenced actions, the Master/Teacher will energetically place Reiki symbols into the student's crown and palms. This action gives the student access to the Universal Life Energy, which he or she can draw upon during the application of Reiki treatments.

Each Reiki Master/Teacher uses his or her own methodology in teaching Reiki classes. Traditionally, each level of Reiki was taught separately. A period of weeks, months, or even years could pass before the Reiki student could go on to the next level. This afforded students time to learn how to use each level proficiently before advancing to the next one. Some Reiki teachers remain true to this tradition. These teachers will only accept a student in their Reiki Level II and Reiki Level III classes when they feel that the student has assimilated the teachings of Level I and Level II, respectively.

Today, you can find almost any combination of Reiki levels taught during one class session. A weekend class could offer both Levels I and II, or even all three levels. The material covered and instructions given may vary somewhat from one classroom to another, but as long as the teacher passes attunements to his or her students, Reiki will become a part of these students forever.

Once Reiki is awakened within you through the attunement ceremony, your journey as a Reiki practitioner begins. You can learn more about Reiki attunements in Chapter 4.

Usui Reiki Level I

Level I is the introductory class to Usui Reiki. In this class, students will receive one, two, or four attunements. The students will learn the history of Reiki, either through listening to the oral tradition or by receiving written handouts that they can take home afterward to read at their leisure. Students will also learn (or review) basic hand placements for giving self-treatments and for treating others. First, the students usually conduct a full-body self-treatment. Then, they may pair off to give and receive a treatment, or the class will participate as a whole in group Reiki treatments.

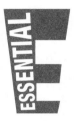

If you have a friend or a relative who shares your interest in Reiki, the two of you may prefer to sign up for a Reiki class together. Using Reiki during and after the class, the two of you will be able to lovingly support one another as you progress with Reiki.

Sign Up for Class

There are a few things to keep in mind when preparing to take your first Reiki class. First, you may be asked to send full payment or a partial deposit a few days or weeks in advance to reserve your place in the class. Often classes are held in people's homes, where the shortness of space might put limits on the class size. This is actually not a disadvantage. Attending a class with only a small number of students, perhaps five or less, can be beneficial in allowing more one-on-one attention between the teacher and students, more time for all of your questions to be answered, and so on. Many individuals who are drawn to learn Reiki are passionate and loving people. Lifetime friendships are likely to develop among the people you will meet in your Reiki classes.

Don't be late for class. Not only does it show poor manners, but it will also inconvenience the teacher by disrupting his well-planned schedule. In such a circumstance, the teacher might either choose to start the class without you, forcing him to help you get caught up later on, or make everyone wait for your arrival before beginning the class, thus possibly inconveniencing other members of the class as well.

Class Preparation

Wear comfortable clothing made of natural fibers such as cotton, wool, or silk. Do not wear nylon stockings or any other restrictive type of garments. And don't forget to eat a good breakfast!

If you are attending a class that will be held out of town, consider reserving a room at a local motel for an overnight stay following your day in class. You will be receiving your attunements and may be participating in three or more full-body treatments. This amounts to a lot of ki energies running through your body.

Attunements by themselves have been known to overwhelm students who are not accustomed to operating on a full tank of energy. Unless you have done some type of energy work prior to your introduction to Reiki, you won't really know how your body will react to that first blast of Reiki energies that surges through it. Some people experience drowsiness or exhaustion, while others feel exhilaration or a sense of loftiness. There are even some students who have reported a sort of buzzing sensation, feeling as if an electric vibrator is running on a high setting right inside his or her body.

Perhaps none of these examples will be representative of your own experience, but should any of them occur, driving home after the class is certainly not a great idea. Even if you believe yourself to be capable of driving, pack an overnight bag to keep in the car with you just in case you do decide later to stop along the way home and spend the night in a motel or with a friend.

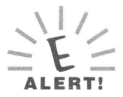

ALERT!

Unless you give plenty of advance notice to your Reiki teacher, don't expect a prepayment or deposit to be refunded if you choose to cancel your class. Advance notice will allow the teacher sufficient time to locate and arrange for another student to take your place.

Basic Class Overview—Reiki Level I

Usually, a basic Reiki Level I class will take somewhere between eight and sixteen hours. Some teachers hold Reiki Level I classes over a two-day period (usually the weekend), while other teachers divide Level I Reiki into two sessions that are held over two consecutive weekends. What follows is a sample syllabus for an eight-hour Reiki Level I class.

Class Schedule

The class will begin at 9:00 A.M. and will go on until 6:00 P.M., including a one-hour break for lunch.

Classroom Introductions

At the beginning of the class, before instruction gets under way, you have a brief period of time to learn your classmates' names and talk informally with your instructor. You may be asked to share something about yourself with the class. For instance, your instructor may ask all the students to state why they are taking the class and what expectations they have, if any.

Class Overview

At the beginning of the class, the teacher may choose to give a formal lecture on Reiki or to facilitate a class discussion about it. Traditionally, this is the time when the "Story of Reiki" is told. The teacher also tells the students what to expect during the class sessions and prompts them to ask any questions they might have before he or she passes the attunements and teaches them the basic hand placements.

Reiki Attunements

The teacher gives basic instructions about how and when attunements are passed. For an all-day class, the passing of attunements could be divided into four short sessions. For example, you might receive two attunements in the morning and two more attunements in the afternoon.

Self-Treatment Instructions

Students are taught the basic hand placements that are used for a full-body self-treatment. Each member of the class gives himself or herself a self-treatment while the teacher supervises.

Instructions for Treating Others

Students are taught the basic hand placements for treating others. To learn, the students practice in pairs, or the teacher may choose to divide them into small groups. Each student should give at least one full-body treatment to another person and receive at least one full-body treatment from someone else.

End of Class

At the end of the class session, you are awarded a certificate for completion of Usui Reiki Level I. Congratulations!

Usui Reiki Level II

Reiki Level II is a continuation of Level I. This level offers the students increased power and the ability to give absentia, or distant, Reiki treatments. In the Reiki Level II class, the teacher will reveal to the students the three Reiki symbols and how they can be used in Reiki treatments. In addition to learning the symbols' meanings, the students will also be able to practice drawing them.

Traditionally, Reiki Level II classes are not available to everyone. Not only does the student need to be already certified as a Reiki Level I practitioner, the instructor must sense that the student is ready to move forward to the next level. Teaching second-degree or third-degree Reiki to a person who isn't psychologically or emotionally ready for it, or is interested in learning Reiki simply for the money or prestige, would be a disservice to Reiki, the student, and the teacher.

Here are a few questions the Reiki Level I practitioner should ask himself or herself before considering going on to Reiki Level II:

- Am I ready for this next step?
- Can I feel Reiki sensations in my palms?
- Do I have a general understanding of Reiki?
- Am I using Reiki on a regular basis?
- What are my reasons for wanting to move on to Reiki Level II?

Basic Class Overview—Reiki Level II

A Reiki Level II class takes approximately six hours to complete and is normally taught in two three-hour sessions, with a break between sessions. It could also be taught in one morning and an afternoon, but it is preferable to teach this class on a weekend, over a two-day period. The following is a sample syllabus for a six-hour Reiki Level II class.

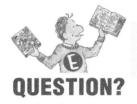

QUESTION?

Why do some Reiki practitioners call themselves "Reiki Sensei"?
Because *sensei* is a Japanese word for "teacher."

Class Schedule

Friday evening: 7:00 P.M. until 10:00 P.M. Saturday morning: 9:00 A.M. until 12:00 P.M.

Introduction Period

Students are given a few minutes to meet and socialize. Typically, students will discuss their individual experiences as Reiki Level I practitioners and their reasons for deciding to take Reiki Level II.

Reiki Level I Review

The teacher gives a brief review of Reiki Level I, and then the students have the opportunity to ask any questions they have concerning Level I and anything else they want to know before they go on to Level II.

Reiki Attunement Rite

The first of two attunements is passed to the students.

Reiki Symbols

The students are introduced to three distinct Reiki symbols (Power, Connection, and Harmony). Students learn how to precisely draw these symbols. They also learn about the power of the symbols and how to pronounce their names and spell them out properly. Sketchpads are provided for the students to use to practice drawing the symbols as they are taught.

Homework Assignment

The Reiki symbols are to be memorized by Saturday morning's class.

Saturday Morning Exam

Students are tested to make sure they can draw the Reiki symbols from memory, recite the symbols' names using correct pronunciations, and know the powers of each symbol.

Reiki Attunement Rite

Second attunement is passed to the students.

Working and Playing with the Symbols

Students learn the absentia Reiki formula and practice sending Reiki treatments to others. The remainder of the class is used to further explore the Reiki symbols. The class may conduct exercises and play games that involve the symbols.

End of Class

The class ends with a brief question-and-answer period. You are awarded a certificate for completion of Usui Reiki Level II. Congratulations!

Teddy Bears and Crayons

Reiki Level II is a fun class to take. The energy level in the classroom is both warm and playful. Remember, everyone in the class is already a Reiki practitioner, so the overall vibes are going to be great! The "memorization" requirement for learning the symbols can feel quite challenging and even a bit stressful for some, but the symbols are really not that difficult to learn. Relax. There is nothing to worry about. If you are struggling with the memorization task, your instructor will be able to help you.

At first you might find a Reiki Level II class to be reminiscent of both an art class and kindergarten class rolled into one. This is because you get to hug teddy bears and draw pictures on art paper with colorful crayons. You might have to be quick to get your hands on the purple crayon before another classmate beats you to it. (Purple is said to naturally carry the vibration of Reiki.) That's why it helps to go to your class fully prepared. Have your own purple marker or crayon tucked inside your pocket or purse. You might also be requested to paint imaginary symbols in the air with your hands. For exercises such as these, Reiki Level II energies will awaken the imaginative powers of the innocent child within you.

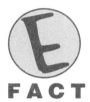

FACT

Purple (or violet) is the color that is commonly associated with carrying Reiki energies. The Japanese word for "purple" is *murasaki* (moo-rah-saa-kee).

The Coveted Reiki Chair

Prior to the arrival of students for her classes, Beverley Jean Voss, Usui Reiki Master, secretly places the Reiki Power symbol into one of the chairs in the living room where she teaches her Reiki classes. During class, she observes how each person naturally gravitates toward that particular seat. Whenever a student gets up from that Reiki-charged chair to go get a cp of tea from the kitchen or to use the bathroom, another student will get up from where he is sitting and plop down into the "hot" chair.

Throughout the class Voss watches amusedly as the chair becomes the coveted seat that everyone wants to sit in—even though none of her students have a clue as to why! Toward the end of the class she finally reveals her earlier clandestine action to the surprise and amusement of her students. Just imagine the reactions—what great fun for all! And what an incredible testament to the power of Reiki symbols!

Usui Reiki Level III

There has always been a bit of confusion about how Reiki III practitioners are different from Reiki Masters and Reiki Master/Teachers. Basically, Reiki Level III is the Reiki Master Level of attunement. Here are the basic distinctions:

- **Reiki Level III**–Title of practitioner who has received the Reiki Master Level attunement.
- **Reiki Master**–Title of practitioner who has received the Reiki Master Level attunement and has been shown the Master symbol.
- **Reiki Master/Teacher**–Title of practitioner who has received the Reiki Master Level attunement, has been shown the Master symbol, and has been taught how to pass attunements to others.

However, these distinctions are somewhat muddied because the title of "Reiki Master" is routinely used by all three categories of practitioners defined in the previous list. Many Master/Teacher practitioners will certify as a "Reiki Master" anyone who has received the Master Level attunement, regardless of whether or not he or she has been given the Master symbol, has learned how to pass attunements, or has received instructions on how to conduct Reiki classes.

When you make the decision to advance from Reiki Level II, it is crucial that you interview several teachers in order to find out what type of training you would receive from them. Also, ask yourself what your motives are for seeking advancement. Are you interested in becoming a teacher and passing on attunements to students? Or are you only trying to receive the Master Level attunement? Unfortunately, some students seek out Master certification only for the sake of title or prestige.

Usui Reiki Master Level

Going through the process of becoming a Reiki Master/Teacher is an intense healing experience on a very personal level. Reiki, as you will learn from going through Reiki Level I and Reiki Level II, brings about balance in your life. Graduation from a Reiki Master Level class does not close the chapter on learning Reiki. Reiki will become an integral part of your life, and learning more about Reiki will continue throughout your lifetime as you use it. The following is a sample syllabus for a Reiki Master/Teacher Level class.

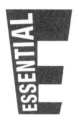

Reiki is not something that can be learned or experienced from a book. Introductory books such as this one are for informational purposes only. They are not meant to serve as a substitute for taking a Reiki class. Readers can use books like this one to learn about the fundamentals of Reiki. Reiki books can also help answer any questions Reiki practitioners may have after taking the classes.

Forty Classroom Hours

Students meet with their instructor for eight-hour class sessions once a week for five weeks. Throughout the course of five weeks, students are instructed to give themselves a full-body self-treatment each day.

First Week

Students and teacher write out goals they hope to achieve in the class. These goals are read out loud every time the class meets. The teacher will present a brief lecture that details the content of the five-week course. Students will be instructed to keep a journal in which they record in detail their personal experiences in the class as well as outside of the classroom. These "experience stories" will be used in their own classes when they start teaching Reiki.

During the class, the teacher will also pass the Master Level attunement to the students and will teach them the Master and Completion symbols. The teacher might end with the following homework assignment: Study history of Reiki. Write down your experience stories. Study instruction handouts for passing first and second attunements for Reiki Level I.

Second Week

The teacher reads aloud the class's goals. Students share their experience stories. The students present the oral history of Dr. Mikao Usui. New experiences since receiving Reiki Master attunement are discussed.

The students learn how to conduct Reiki Level I classes and review how to pass first and second attunements for Reiki Level I. The following would be assigned for homework: Continue to add experience stories to your list. Review the history of Reiki. Practice the attunement process. Study instruction handouts for passing third and fourth attunements for Reiki Level I. Memorize all Reiki symbols, including the Master and Completion symbols.

Third Week

Again, the teacher reviews the goals by reading them out loud, and students share their experience stories. Then, students present the oral history of Dr. Hayashi.

Students review how to pass third and fourth attunements for Reiki Level I. Reiki Level II class structure is discussed. Students are tested on all the symbols (how to draw, pronounce, and interpret them). As a homework assignment, students may be required to study instructional handouts on passing attunements for Reiki Level II and review the history of Reiki.

Fourth Week

After the overview of the class goals and sharing experience stories, students present the oral history of Mrs. Hawayo Takata. Then, students go over how to pass attunements for Reiki Level II. Reiki Level II class structure is also reviewed. Classroom and Reiki Master ethics are discussed. The homework assignment is to study instructional handouts for passing Master Level attunements.

Fifth Week

The last class begins in the usual manner, with the reading of goals, followed by students sharing their experience stories. Then, students go over how to pass attunements for Reiki Master Level and the class structure of the Reiki Master Level class.

End of Class

The class ends with a brief question-and-answer period. You are awarded a certificate for completion of Usui Reiki Master Level. Congratulations!

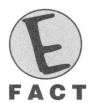

FACT

At the end of the Reiki Level III class, students review passing attunements for all levels. Additional classes are scheduled for any students who feel that they may need more instruction.

What It All Means

Certifications in the various levels of Reiki are paper documents noting participation and accomplishment in classroom studies. In the end, the surest way to develop a true mastering of Reiki is through practicing it routinely, applying the five Reiki Principles, and involving Reiki in every aspect of your daily life.

Reiki I is the awakening. Reiki II is intended to increase the students' power and to teach them how to assist others by learning how to do distant healings. Reiki III and Master Levels are intended to teach students the skills needed to teach and pass attunements to others. A distinctive attunement ritual is passed from teacher to student at each level.

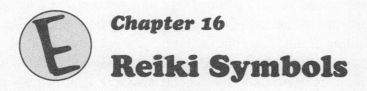

Chapter 16

Reiki Symbols

There are five symbols used in the Usui Reiki attunement process. Four of these symbols are also used in conducting both hands-on and distant treatments. There is much mystery surrounding the Reiki symbols because of the tradition to honor their sacredness and to guard them from the eyes of nonpractitioners. The development, definitions, purposes, and methods of using the Reiki symbols are subjects of great interest and discussion.

The Power of a Symbol

Through Hawayo Takata's Reiki stories, her students were taught that the Reiki symbols were revealed to Dr. Mikao Usui through spiritual enlightenment on the twenty-first day of his meditation fast on Mt. Kurama. According to Takata, Usui had recognized these symbols from his studies of the ancient Sanskrit writings kept in the monastery's libraries, but before his spiritual awakening on the mountain, he supposedly had no understanding of the meanings or the purpose of these symbols.

However, no definite proof that Usui actually reviewed or studied any Sanskrit documents has ever come to light. Also, the Reiki symbols employed by Usui are formulated from Chinese and Japanese kanji characters, not Sanskrit lettering. Usui either developed the Reiki symbols on his own, or he may have translated them from the ethereal knowledge revealed to him on the mountain by using his own written language, Japanese kanji.

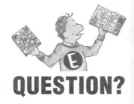

QUESTION?

From where did kanji originate?
Kanji are modified Chinese characters, originally imported from China. In addition to its use of kanji, the Japanese writing system also relies on hiragana and katakana, alphabetic systems that represent various sounds, as opposed to ideas or words.

Japanese Kanji

For the Japanese, a handwritten kanji is a character equivalent to a written letter, word, or phrase in Western handwriting. Kanji characters are pictograms that represent ideas or words, rather than merely alphabet letters or syllables of words that you would sound out in order to read. Whereas the word "Reiki" consists of five letters in the English alphabet, in Japanese writings Reiki is pictured as a "kanji-pair." In other words, Reiki is represented by two individual kanji symbols, often drawn one on top of the other. The top symbol is *rei,* meaning "universal life," and the lower symbol is *ki,* meaning "energy."

Before the invention of typewriters and computers with Japanese fonts, the Japanese wrote their characters with a paintbrush or pen. There are many versions of "Reiki kanji," mainly because of the differences in people's handwriting styles. Modified kanji characters are now available as fonts in computer software programs.

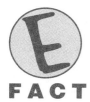

FACT

Modern Japanese–English dictionaries have quite a few translations for the word "Reiki": 1) sacred ground; 2) established rule; 3) chill, cold weather; 4) electrical excitation; 5) aura; 6) healing method.

The Five Reiki Symbols

However he derived them, Usui used the five Reiki symbols as practical teaching tools for his students—the symbols were meant to assist the students in focusing and holding intention while giving treatments and passing attunements.

Five Traditional Reiki Symbols			
Japanese Name	**English Name**	**Intention**	**Purposes**
Cho Ku Rei	Power symbol	Light switch	Manifestation; increased power; accelerated healing; healing catalyst
Sei Hei Ki	Harmony symbol	Purification	Cleansing; protection; mental and emotional healing
Hon Sha Ze Sho Nen	Connection symbol	Timelessness	Distant healing; past/present/future; healing karma; spiritual connection
Dai Ko Myo	Master symbol	Enlightenment	Empowerment; soul healing; oneness
Raku	Completion symbol	Grounding	Kundalini healing; hara connection; chakra alignment

Imagery Is a Universal Language

Energy, in its purest essence, does not possess "form," nor is it visually identifiable. However, in the physical world in which we live, the concept of visualizing or touching a structured energy form is often easier to comprehend than visualizing manipulation of shapeless or invisible energy. Usui's symbols became visual representations of "all that Reiki is." Usui understood that Reiki was a universal energy. Usui not only was able to give the symbols to his students as healing tools, but, through graphic images, he managed to give Reiki its own universal language.

Imagery truly is a universal language, eye-candy for our visual pleasure. Everyday pictures, icons, and symbols are used in our communications to represent our ideas and inspirations. When they are viewed, certain images can signify clear-cut meanings. There are many examples, such as a glowing light bulb to symbolize a bright idea, the skull and crossbones to warn of poisonous contents, a red heart to indicate love, and the four-leaf clover to suggest good fortune. When we see these easily recognizable images, their associated meanings come to our minds instantly.

When practitioners use Reiki symbols regularly, they soon learn that the power is not in the symbols themselves, but in the purposes and intentions they represent and solidify.

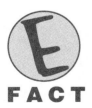

FACT

Emoticons are facial expressions represented on a computer screen with certain combinations of punctuation marks. Internet users have come to rely on emoticons to convey their feelings in personal e-mails and while chatting online. Most often, emoticons depict the image of a face, flipped ninety degrees.

E-mail Emoticons

E-mail emoticons help us express our emotions and intentions when communicating with others via the Internet. When a sentence or phrase in an e-mail communication is followed by an emoticon, it helps the recipient of your e-mail to better understand what mood you are in at the time you type your message.

- Smiley face   :-)
- Frowny face   :-(
- Angelic look   O:-)
- Surprised look   =O
- Confused look   %-(
- Sticking out tongue :-P
- Wink   ;-)

What do emoticons have to do with Reiki symbols? Emoticons are images that convey a person's "intent" when delivering a message. Using Reiki symbols is also a means to express one's "intent." When conducting Reiki treatments, employing the Reiki symbols affords the practitioner a focal point for his or her healing intentions.

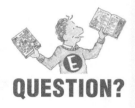

QUESTION?

Who invented the smiley face emoticon?
Computer science professor Scott E. Fahlman created the "smiley" emoticon on September 19, 1982. Fahlman suggested that the character string :-), when read sideways in an online communication, could indicate that a comment was not meant to be taken seriously.

Shrouded in Secrecy

Reiki symbols are not available to everyone. Reiki students are introduced to the first three symbols after they are attuned to Reiki Level II. Those who go on to the Reiki Master/Teacher Level are taught the two remaining symbols. An introduction to Reiki symbols includes learning how to draw them and instruction as to what they mean and how they may be used in Reiki.

Traditionally, any drawings of the Reiki symbols on paper were burned in a ritual at the end of the classes. Sometimes this ritual would be a part of the class. At other times the teacher would perform a private ritual, burning the drawings after the students were gone. Modern teachers who still honor the tradition of keeping the symbols private will either burn the drawings or use a paper shredder so that the paper waste can later be recycled. Other teachers see no harm in allowing students to keep their classroom drawings and may even provide predrawn diagrams in handouts that the students can keep for future reference.

One reason for keeping the symbols hidden was to prevent the powers within the symbols from being misused if they fell into the wrong hands. This reasoning seems to contradict the premise that Reiki does no harm. Today, diagrams of the Reiki symbols can be readily found printed in books and on the Internet. However, there is still controversy among Reiki practitioners over whether or not these symbols should be kept private. You can read more about Reiki controversies in Chapter 20.

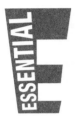

Whenever any Reiki symbol is to be used, the practitioner recites it three times. This may be done aloud or mentally, as the practitioner traces the symbol in the air over the recipient's body.

Cho Ku Rei—the Power Symbol

The Reiki Power symbol is the first symbol presented to Reiki initiates; it is the most commonly used Reiki symbol. In fact, it is used more often than all the other symbols combined.

Reiki practitioners use the Cho Ku Rei symbol by itself or in combination with the other symbols. When conducting a distant treatment, using two Power symbols as energetic bookends with a Connection symbol sandwiched in between creates a power-packed vacuum space that will travel at lightning speed. When the treatment is delivered, the results can be immediate and far-reaching.

From a Visual Perspective

When you draw the symbols on paper, they will appear flat and lifeless. However, if you draw them in the air, they evolve into three-dimensional animated images. It is as if the ki energies breathe life into them. The symbols will float in the air as if they are hanging from a mobile. They will shrink and enlarge and even change colors. As one Reiki Level II practitioner described it, "I visualize a Japanese man drawing the symbols on a chalkboard. I then visualize the chalk-drawn symbols peeling off the board and lifting up into the air." The symbols will float across the room where she is sitting while conducting a full-body treatment on a client. From there she will manipulate the symbols either mentally or with her hands, as needed.

Purrs Like a Kitten

The Power symbol is a wonderful catalyst for the healing process. If you have ever held a purring kitten, you will understand the "motor" vibration associated with the Cho Ku Rei. There is an underlying current or charge that resides in the core of the coil of this symbol. The strength of this charge may be subtle at times and revved up high at other times, but even though the energy embedded within the symbol may cool down or unwind, it always maintains a constant pulse.

You can draw the Cho Ku Rei with as many spiral movements as you feel are appropriate for the situation at hand. Printed diagrams of the Cho Ku Rei normally show two and a half coils, but you can draw the Cho Ku Rei with as many coils as you like. Don't worry about winding up any coil too tightly, and be sure to draw the coils, or spirals, counterclockwise.

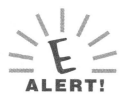
ALERT!

Controversy continues to persist in the Reiki community today as to whether or not the Reiki symbols should be kept private or drawn openly and made available for anyone and everyone to see and use.

Metaphysical Multiplier

The primary intention of using the Cho Ku Rei is to increase power. This is why it is praised for its manifestation power. It is a metaphysical multiplier. No matter what aspect of your life you desire to increase, Reiki's Power symbol is an intention tool that can help bring it to fruition. There are many areas in your life that can benefit from the boost of energy provided by the Cho Ku Rei. Listed here are just some of the effects this symbol can have:

- Bolster self-confidence
- Increase cash flow
- Expand time
- Actualize dreams
- Intensify creativity
- Boost immune system
- Promote spiritual growth
- Magnify happiness

Sei Hei Ki—the Harmony Symbol

The Reiki Harmony symbol is the second symbol Reiki initiates learn in their Level II class. This symbol is used as a purification tool and is also helpful to anyone dealing with emotional or mental disturbances. This is the symbol that assists a person who is trying to break a simple bad habit or overcome the grip of a serious physiological or mental addiction.

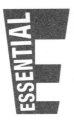

The Sei Hei Ki symbol works very well in combination with Bach's Rescue Remedy flower essence formula in both first-aid and trauma situations. Rescue Remedy is a combination of five individual essences that is used for treating symptoms of anxiety and shock. It helps stabilize trauma situations by restoring a person's state of calm and confidence.

Like a Fire-Breathing Dragon

The Sei Hei Ki looks remarkably like a cartoon dragon. Cartoon dragons are not to be feared. Rather, they should be understood and enjoyed as friendly and courageous beings.

Nevertheless, the Reiki dragon is up to the challenge when faced with fighting off adversity. Although the symbol does not show the dragon's fiery breath, you can easily add it in your imagination. The fire essence within the Sei Hei Ki serves as a purification flame. It scorches addictions and expels negative energies, leaving nothing but smoldering ashes upon the ground, allowing the rebirth of energy in its purest form.

A Personal Bodyguard

In addition to its label as the Harmony symbol, the Sei Hei Ki is also often named the Protection symbol. In its protective capacity, the Sei Hei Ki can be used as an antiseptic "ointment" before, during, and after surgery. It can also be applied as a protective shield prior to and following purification ceremonies or whenever menacing energies have been removed from the auric field or physical body.

Sei Hei Ki can be used in prayer mantras when asking for personal protection and safe travel conditions before driving, flying, taking a vacation cruise, and so on. The Sei Hei Ki symbol can be placed inside packages as additional insurance for their safe delivery before dropping them off at the post office. This Protection symbol can even be placed in condoms as an extra precaution before indulging in "safe sex."

As with all protective measures, there is no guarantee that using the Sei Hei Ki will be 100 percent effective. If it's in the cards, a traffic accident or pregnancy could still occur, no matter how many precautions have been taken. However, using the Sei Hei Ki as a cautionary intention in your day-to-day existence is recommended. After all, would you go out without wearing an overcoat if a heavy rainstorm was in the forecast? Of course you wouldn't. The Sei Hei Ki is an added protective covering to help you weather the stormy elements of life.

Hon Sha Ze Sho Nen—the Connection Symbol

The Reiki Connection symbol is the third symbol taught to Reiki initiates. The Hon Sha Ze Sho Nen is best known for its use in distant, or absentia, treatments. This symbol has a long reach; it extends beyond time and space. This symbol is also called "the Pagoda" because of its towerlike appearance. Multiple kanji characters are used to create it. More variations have been shown of this symbol than any of the other Reiki symbols.

From a visual point of view, the Hon Sha Ze Sho Nen is a cosmic shape-shifter. This symbol is extremely adaptable and feels elastic when you work with it. Its form collapses and stretches, as needed, in any application. More so than the other symbols, the Hon Sha Ze Sho Nen seems to exhibit extra flexibility.

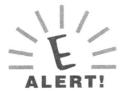

ALERT!

All the Reiki symbols are flexible. Working with these symbols could be described as handling modeling clay. Clay sculptures express what the artist feels. In this same way, the Reiki symbols emulate intentions put forth by the Reiki practitioner.

Absentia Treatments

The Hon Sha Ze Sho Nen is always used in transmitting absentia, or distant, treatments. It possesses the power of telepathy and is comparable to the electrical wiring that connects telegraph operators on each end of a communication. You can read more about this symbol and distant treatments in Chapter 8, which describes absentia treatments in more detail.

Inner-Child Therapy

The Hon Sha Ze Sho Nen can assist you in making a connection with your inner child. Unresolved childhood traumas and issues tend to get buried inside our subconscious minds, contributing to our adult fears and concerns. Reiki treatments can bring about balance and will sometimes bring these issues to the surface for healing. When practitioners encounter hurtful memories that were formerly locked up inside a recipient but are suddenly beginning to surface, it is appropriate to apply this symbol to assist the ki movement toward balance and healing.

Akashic Records

The Connection symbol serves as the key to accessing information recorded in the Akashic Records (see Appendix B for more information on the Akashic Records). This information is included for individuals who believe in reincarnation. If you believe that you have lived many lifetimes, you probably also believe that when you entered your current incarnation, you brought in talents and knowledge that you attained during previous incarnations. Also, any emotional backlash from pains or sufferings that were not completely healed would also have been carried in at birth.

There's one school of thought that teaches the belief that all of our lifetimes (past, present, and future) are being lived out simultaneously in different dimensions. The Hon Sha Ze Sho Nen symbol can extend to past and future lives and treat all dis-eases from all our lifetimes. Applying Reiki to ailments that originated from previous lifetimes will treat the physical dis-ease during that lifetime, and, as a bonus, it will also treat any lingering emotional repercussions that were carried over into your present lifetime.

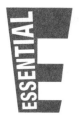

When visualizing the Reiki symbols, pay attention to whether or not they appear balanced. A symbol that appears askew is signaling an imbalance. For example, if you're conducting a distant treatment and the Cho Ku Rei appears lopsided, it could mean that the recipient's personal power is diminished. Or, if the Sei Hei Ki appears squashed, it could indicate disharmony. In these cases, ask your Reiki guides to bring balance to the misaligned symbol before sending it off to the recipient.

Dai Ko Myo—the Master Symbol

The Master symbol is possibly the single most coveted Reiki symbol by first- and second-degree practitioners. This is because most people are achievement-oriented. We want to earn the highest badge or be awarded the grandest trophy.

The energy represented by the Reiki Master symbol is powerful. It represents *all that is Reiki,* including love and personal empowerment. This is why the Master symbol is included in all levels of attunement. All levels of Reiki practitioners receive the Dai Ko Myo symbol from their teacher through the attunement ritual. It is not an exclusive energy available only to some people; Dai Ko Myo love energy is accessible to everyone.

Being attuned to Reiki Master Level and knowing how to draw the Master symbol are required for teachers in order for them to be able to attune others. But, aside from that, the symbol is seldom, if ever, used. The symbol can be drawn or visualized in healings, but the essence of this symbol is already in the energy of Reiki itself. Probably the only time it might be called upon is whenever you are treating someone who is struggling with self-love.

Raku—the Completion Symbol

The last Reiki symbol in the Usui Reiki system is the Raku. This symbol is used only in the final stage of the attunement ritual in order to separate the teacher's aura from his or her student's aura. Its energy is very forceful and should carefully be placed between the two individuals.

Aside from being used to separate the auras and align the student's chakras, the Raku has no other use in Reiki. Its appearance is that of a sharp zigzag image that resembles a lightning bolt. The Raku is drawn from top to bottom. An alternate Raku symbol, occasionally used by nontraditional Reiki Masters, resembles a winding snake and represents Kundalini energy.

Meditation and Reiki Symbols

Each symbol carries its own unique energy and has distinct purposes. Once you learn a symbol, spend some time with it individually in order to form a close relationship with it. The symbols are wonderful healing tools, but trying to use them without knowing their full potential or understanding how or when to utilize them will diminish your awareness of the healing process. Meditate on each symbol individually and take note of any sensations and thoughts that surface.

The Reiki symbols are very beautiful, but they have no power by themselves. They are merely visual representatives of all that Reiki has to offer. They serve as tools to assist Reiki practitioners when shaping their healing intentions during self-treatments and whenever treating others. Each practitioner develops his or her own unique relationship with the symbols.

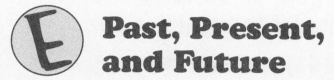

Chapter 17

Past, Present, and Future

Reiki initiates continue to explore Reiki's historical past and its enduring development into the present day. From where did Reiki originate? How did it make its way from the Far East to the Western Hemisphere? Why are there so many variations in the stories told about Reiki's history? Is the healing art that is being taught today, Usui Reiki, an incomplete version of the original teachings? These are just a few of the questions being raised about the origins and current teachings of Reiki.

Usui Reiki Emerges in the West

Usui Shiki Ryoho Reiki arrived in Hawaii from Japan through the efforts of a Japanese-American Reiki Master named Hawayo Takata. In 1937, Hawayo Takata moved from Hawaii to the mainland of the United States. Before her death in 1980, she initiated twenty-two Masters from among her many Reiki students. From these twenty-two individuals, Reiki has branched out far and wide across the globe.

The Story of Hawayo Takata

It is fortunate that Hawayo Takata was interested in learning how Reiki worked, or Reiki may have never made its way from Japan to the West. Hawayo Takata played a major role in helping spread Reiki to all corners of the globe. Following is a retelling of the story of how Hawayo Takata became interested in the workings of Reiki.

Hawayo Takata was very ill and was scheduled to undergo surgery to improve her health. As she prepared for surgery, she heard a voice telling her that surgery was not necessary and that there was another way to be cured. She asked around the surgical hospital where she was admitted what other remedies were available to her and someone told her about Reiki. She left the hospital and sought out Dr. Chujiro Hayashi's Reiki clinic in Japan.

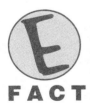

FACT

Hawayo Takata received her Reiki Level I and II training in Tokyo, Japan, in 1936 and 1937 from Chujiro Hayashi. In 1938, Hayashi visited Hawayo Takata's homeland of Hawaii and initiated her as a Reiki Master/Teacher.

Hawayo Takata soon found herself lying upon a table to receive her first full-body Reiki treatment as an alternative to having surgery. When one of the practitioners placed his hands on her, she could feel the vibrational flow and heat from the Reiki pouring out from the practitioner's palms. She believed there must have been some mechanism that was activating the impulses she was experiencing. She looked up the sleeve of his garment to investigate but saw that nothing was there. She marveled that such an outpouring of energy was happening without the use of a device of some kind. She experienced profound healing from Reiki and made it her life path to learn more about Reiki.

Historical Truth or Aesop Fable?

When Takata began teaching Reiki to her students, she incorporated storytelling as a teaching aid to instill Reiki values. The stories of Hawayo Takata, in which she described to her students how Dr. Mikao Usui rediscovered Reiki, became a core component in the teachings of Reiki in the West.

It turns out that the stories Hawayo Takata told about the history of Reiki, stories that were subsequently passed down from teacher to student, were not altogether accurate. For one reason or another, Hawayo Takata deliberately peppered them with certain embellishments that stretched the truth. There has been much speculation as to why Hawayo Takata might have felt the need to color her Reiki stories. One theory is that she never intended for them to be taken literally, as historical truths, but rather as metaphors or parables that teach certain moral codes for living your life in the Reiki way. It may be that her stories were meant not only to teach the fundamentals of Reiki but also to inspire moral conduct and instill ethical values in her students.

The Oral Tradition

One aspect of Takata's stories that turned out to be untrue in the literal sense was her claim that the stories she told had always been passed down through the oral tradition. Students were instructed not to write down or otherwise record Takata's Reiki stories or teachings. The Reiki stories, five principles, sacred symbols, and attunement procedures were to be locked up and preserved only within the minds of Reiki practitioners. In this way, they would forever remain shielded from the prying eyes of nonpractitioners. Practitioners were taught that protection of the knowledge of Reiki and the secrecy of the Reiki symbols were of the utmost importance.

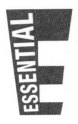

Instructional manuals of both of Takata's predecessors, Dr. Mikao Usui and Chujiro Hayashi, have since surfaced in Japan and, although not confirmed, it is possible that these texts were actually dispensed as "handbooks" to their Reiki students.

Other Myths

One story that circulated among Reiki initiates in the West claimed that at one time Mikao Usui attended college in Chicago, Illinois. Despite careful background checks into the life of Usui, this information has never been substantiated. Furthermore, research by Frank Arjava Petter helped to dispel the accounts that suggested Usui was a practicing Christian. It has been suggested that certain elements in the Reiki stories were fabricated in order to make the practice of Reiki more palatable for students who were of the Christian faith.

Western students were also informed that all the Japanese Reiki practitioners either died during World War II or that, after hiding in the hills during that era for fear of retribution, they never returned to the populated areas to pass on Reiki's teachings to others. And yet, Reiki flourishes in Japan today.

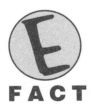

In different versions of Reiki stories, Dr. Mikao Usui has been portrayed in a variety of roles. In some stories, he is represented as a medical doctor, in others as professor of theology, Buddhist scholar, Christian monk, priest, minister, and spiritualist.

Takata may very well have been selective in deciding which aspects of Reiki she would teach her Western students. Clearly, she omitted some of the more spiritual components that she had learned while studying Reiki in Japan with Chujiro Hayashi. The regimented Reiki hand placements were not part of Usui's teachings. Usui taught Reiki as a spiritual way of life and an intuitive healing art, allowing the practitioner's intuition to direct hand placements during a treatment. The organized hand placements were added into the system later, either by Hayashi or Takata. The use of the basic hand placements proved to be a practical tool for beginners.

Reiki Stories Retold

Another explanation for the discrepancies in Hawayo Takata's stories is that Takata may have told the stories somewhat differently each time she recounted them. Furthermore, it's not clear how much of the stories related by Takata's initiates to their students were retold as precisely as Takata had communicated them. It's possible that subsequent retellings of the Reiki stories distorted their content even more as they were passed down orally from teacher to student.

Did you ever play the game of "telephone" or "gossip" as a child? If so, you will recall sitting in a circle on the floor with a group of your friends. The first person would whisper a sentence to the person sitting next to her. In turn, that person would pass on what was said to the next person sitting on the other side. The whispered sentence would continue to get repeated to the next person in the circle and so on until, finally, at the end of the game, the very last person would state out loud what message was whispered to him. As almost always happens, this final message would be very different from the original, and everyone would giggle with glee.

This child's game is a good illustration of how it came to be that so many different versions of Reiki's history have come to light. Because the stories were never written down, they were continually modified as they were passed down orally.

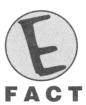

FACT

The tradition among Usui Reiki Masters to orate the Reiki stories to their students continues even today. Some teachers never question the validity of the tales and will tell the stories to their students in much the same way as they themselves heard them from their own teachers. Others do so with a reminder to their students that the stories have many versions and that it will be up to them to judge what is true and what is fiction.

The Tale of Rediscovery

One of the stories Hawayo Takata told her students had to do with how Reiki was "rediscovered" by a Japanese man named Mikao Usui. The story describes the rediscovery as the result of Usui's spiritual quest to learn about the miracle of hands-on healing that was used by both Jesus Christ and Buddha. According to the story, Usui turned away from his secular life and interviewed religious luminaries of the period in search of this knowledge. He also conducted extensive research of Sanskrit writings as he continued to look for answers. But it was not until he put the books away and spent several days fasting and meditating that he became "inspired" and Reiki was revealed to him. The following is one version of the story.

A Question of Theology

Dr. Mikao Usui was a learned man who was a college professor of theology. During one of his classroom lectures, a student asked him if he believed the passage of Bible scripture where Jesus told his disciples that all men could perform miraculous healings by laying on hands. Usui's response was that he believed it to be true. Then the student asked Dr. Usui to give a demonstration. But Usui was not able to give the demonstration. Although he believed it to be true, he did not know how to heal with his hands.

Shortly afterward, Dr. Usui resigned from his teaching position at the Japanese college and began a quest to find the answer to his student's question. His travels took him far into India and Tibet. He spent many years in a Buddhist monastery toiling over Sanskrit scrolls, becoming increasingly frustrated because he didn't have enough understanding of Sanskrit to translate what he was reading. Feeling defeated, he sought out the monastery's abbot for counsel. The abbot suggested that he go on retreat to a mountaintop and do a twenty-one-day meditation fast.

Meditation on the Mountain

On the mountaintop, Usui counted out twenty-one stones and placed them in a pile. Each morning at dawn he would take one of the stones and toss it away. Each day he waited for inspiration, but nothing came. On the twenty-first morning, after he had tossed his final stone, Usui threw his body face down onto the ground and sobbed because he had not been given any answers and would make his journey back down the mountain later that day without knowing any more than he did before he started. Then, as he sat upright on the mountaintop, he felt something strike him on his forehead, where his third-eye chakra was located, and he fainted. After regaining consciousness, he opened his eyes and saw bubbles of purple light floating toward him. It was at this moment that Usui was given the knowledge of Reiki. The Reiki symbols were defined in gold letters inside the floating bubbles. Not only did he see the symbols, but he also became aware of their meanings and how to use them for healing. Usui had his answer, and he couldn't wait to share his finding with the abbot.

Three Miracles

As Usui scurried down the mountainside, he stubbed his toe and tore his toenail. After he applied Reiki energies to his injured toe, the bleeding stopped and his toe was healed. At the bottom of the mountain Usui stopped by a roadside table where a family living nearby prepared small, inexpensive meals to passing travelers. Usui sat down at their roadside table and requested a full meal. The man told Usui that he should not eat so much after fasting for so many days. His concern was that Usui would become ill. He said he would prepare Usui some rice gruel. However, Usui insisted on a larger meal, assuring the man that his body would be able to digest it without problem.

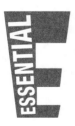

Dr. Mikao Usui experienced three healing miracles shortly after rediscovering Reiki: He healed his stubbed toe, he cured the farmer's granddaughter's toothache, and he had no trouble eating a full meal following a twenty-one-day fast.

When the man's granddaughter delivered the meal to him, Usui noticed that she had a cloth wrapped around her head and chin. When he asked her about it, the young girl told Usui that she suffered from a toothache and, unfortunately, the doctor of the region would not be traveling their way for several days. Dr. Usui then offered to place his hands on the young girl's jaw to heal her toothache. After agreeing to let him do this, both the girl and her grandfather were amazed at the healing and very pleased with the results. Usui finished his large meal without any digestive problems. The man would not accept any monetary payment for the meal, insisting that his granddaughter's healing would be gratefully accepted in exchange for the meal.

Bedridden Abbot

After returning to the monastery, Usui discovered that the abbot was very ill and had been bedridden for several days. After Usui was ushered into the abbot's bedroom, he placed his hands on him. The arthritic abbot was immediately able to get out of bed and walk about the room without feeling any stiffness or soreness. Healing the abbot was Usui's fourth Reiki miracle.

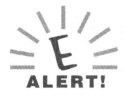

ALERT!

"Every religion emphasizes human improvement, love, respect for others, sharing other people's suffering. On these lines every religion has more or less the same viewpoint and the same goal."

—THE DALAI LAMA

Administering Reiki in Tokyo

Usui spent the next several years in a poor district of Tokyo, administering Reiki to the crippled and sick beggars that filled its streets. Many healing miracles occurred. After a while, Usui noticed that some of the individuals he had healed in the earlier years were returning to the streets as beggars. He asked them why they weren't working at jobs and improving their standard of living. They told him that it was too difficult for them to work, that it was easier to live as beggars. Usui realized that he had healed only the physical ailments of these people.

Dr. Usui knew that in order for Reiki to reach its full potential, it had to heal emotional, spiritual, and mental imbalances as well. He therefore left the slums and began working on the spiritual precepts that have come to be known as the Reiki Precepts. He also realized that in order for Reiki to be valued, there must be some type of energy exchange.

The Reiki Creed

The moral codes that Reiki practitioners are advised to incorporate into their Reiki practice are called the Reiki Precepts (Gokai). These codes are intended as words to live by each day. They are aligned with most other religions' basic moralistic principle—that it is responsible and virtuous for people to care for one another.

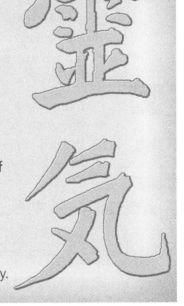

Mikao Usui's Reiki Precepts

The secret of inviting happiness through many
    blessings
The spiritual medicine for all illness

For today only: Do not anger

For today only: Do not worry

For today only: Be humble

For today only: Be honest in your work

For today only: Be compassionate to yourself
    and others

Do Gassho every morning and evening.
Keep in your mind and recite.

Usui Reiki Ryoho—Improve your mind and body.

Original Intent of the Precepts

Mikao Usui taught his students to recite the precepts twice daily, once in the morning and again in the evening. While reciting the precepts, the practitioner's hands were held in prayer (in the Gassho Position). These precepts were also to be recited silently prior to the empowerment (attunement) ceremony, whenever a new student was initiated as a Reiki practitioner.

The intent of the precepts is to assist Reiki practitioners in breaking away from the bad habit of reverting to past experiences and instead to focus on the present. We cannot change the past. Nor is it productive to be overly concerned about our future. But we can do better today. Usui's precepts urge the practitioner to become consciously aware of the present day.

The Reiki Principles are also intended to help us recognize that our emotions and anxieties do not promote healing. We need to let go of our frustrations and concerns and focus on living simply, being reliable and useful to others and gentle with ourselves, and showing kindness to others—and our lives will be the better for it. The application of the Reiki Principles helps us to be mindful of our reactions; it conditions us not to react in a negative way but rather to be appreciative of the people around us and of the simple things in life.

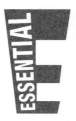

Extinguishing anger is very different from repressing it. Feelings of anger should never be ignored and should always be validated. But expressing the feelings in a way that disrupts harmony in your life is certainly not the Reiki way.

Additional Versions of Usui's Precepts

One can only speculate as to why Hayashi chose to rewrite Usui's precepts in his own words and rename them "ideals" and, in turn, why Takata adapted Hayashi's ideals into her differently worded "principles." Differences in the exact wordings appear to have happened naturally. Their versions do not detract from the original purpose set forth by Dr. Usui; they are merely expressed somewhat differently. All of these represent the essential moral framework that is fostered by respectable and principled practitioners.

Reiki practitioners may choose to adopt Usui's Reiki Precepts, Hayashi's Reiki Ideals, or Takata's Principles. Optionally, they may choose to modify the words in a manner that suits them, as long as the basic meanings remain comparable. Dozens of variations of Usui's five Reiki Precepts have been developed.

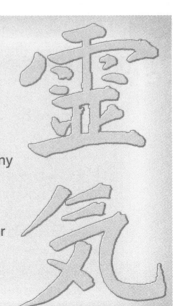

Dr. Hayashi's Five Ideals

Just for today: Do not worry.

Just for today: Do not anger.

Just for today: Honor your teachers, your father and mother, and your neighbors; count your blessings; and show appreciation for your food.

Just for today: Earn your living honestly.

Just for today: Be kind to everything that has life.

Hawayo Takata's Principles

Just for today, I will not be angry.

Just for today, I will not worry.

Just for today, I will give thanks for my many blessings.

Just for today, I will do my work honestly.

Just for today, I will be kind to my neighbor and every living thing.

Researching Reiki's Japanese Roots

Recently, Reiki practitioners like Frank Arjava Petter, William Lee Rand, Walter Lübeck, and Hiroshi Doi have been visiting Japan with the hope of unraveling the mysteries surrounding the true history of Reiki. A wealth of information has come to light through their investigative actions and their interviews with people living in Japan. Around the mid-1990s, these investigators began publishing works that detailed the findings of their research, making the information available to the general public. Following are some of the conclusions that they have made based on their findings.

Dr. Usui's complete first name is Mikaomi Usui. During his lifetime, he founded a society in Japan named Usui Reiki Ryoho Gakkai. This society is still in existence today. Usui's Reiki Precepts originated from Meiji Emperor's five rules for life. After his death, Usui was buried in Tokyo's Saihoji Temple Cemetery. At the cemetery, you can still view the memorial stone erected in his honor.

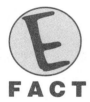

FACT

The terms *master* and *grand master* were never used in Japan. Takata invented the use of the term *master* as an English translation for the highest level of Usui Reiki training, or Shinpiden, a Japanese term that may be translated as "mystery," not "mastery."

Chujiro Hayashi was only one of at least sixteen individuals who received the highest level of Reiki attunements and training from Usui. Furthermore, Hayashi may have been the last person to receive Shinpiden (Master Level) from Usui, since the documented date of his initiation is one year prior to Usui's death. Eventually, Hayashi broke away from the Usui Reiki Ryoho Gakkai, created his own form of Reiki, and established a Reiki clinic known as the Hayashi Reiki Institute. Hayashi's successor was his wife, Chie Hayashi. Mrs. Hayashi continued to practice Reiki in Japan after World War II.

Japanese Reiki practitioners who are associated with Usui Reiki Ryoho Gakkai are an exclusive and private group. Most of the Reiki practitioners who practice in Japan today learned Reiki from Western teachers.

Usui Shiki Ryoho Timeline

All of the information that has been learned about the history of Reiki in Japan, plus the more recent history of how it developed and spread all over the world, may be organized into a timeline of events:

1922: Dr. Mikao Usui develops Reiki following an inspiration he received during a fasting meditation. He founds a society in Japan that he names Usui Reiki Ryoho Gakkai.

1925: Dr. Hayashi receives Shinpiden (Reiki Master Level) from Dr. Usui.

1926: Dr. Mikao Usui suffers a stroke and dies.

1936: Mrs. Hawayo Takata attunes to Shoden (Reiki Level I) from Dr. Hayashi.

1937: Mrs. Hawayo Takata attains Okuden (Reiki Level II) and returns to her home in Hawaii.

1938: Mrs. Hawayo Takata receives Shinpiden (Reiki Master Level) from Dr. Hayashi. She establishes two Reiki clinics in Hawaii.

1941: Dr. Chujiro Hayashi passes away.

1976: Mrs. Hawayo Takata begins initiating students to Reiki Master Level.

1978: Mrs. Hawayo Takata attunes Barbara Weber Ray to Reiki Master Level.

1979: Phyllis Lei Furumoto is attuned to Reiki Master Level.

1980: Mrs. Hawayo Takata dies. By the time of her death, she had initiated twenty-two students to Reiki Master Level, including her granddaughter Phyllis Lei Furumoto and her sister Kay Yamashita.

1980: Barbara Weber Ray founds the American Reiki Association, Inc. (later renamed the Radiance Technique International Association, Inc.). Ray declares herself to be Takata's successor.

1983: The Reiki Alliance is founded. Phyllis Lei Furumoto is named Reiki Grand Master, successor to Hawayo Takata.

1997: Phyllis Lei Furumoto and the Reiki Alliance attempt to trademark the words *Reiki* and *Usui Shiki Ryoho*. The trademark application is denied.

1998–present: Reiki continues to evolve.

For more historical information on the various roles played by Usui, Hayashi, Takata, Takata's twenty-two students, and other Reiki Masters, see Chapter 18.

Evolution of Reiki

The reasons why some Reiki stories were fabricated and certain modifications were made to the teaching materials made available to Takata's students may never be fully understood. But in spite of the false facts and misleading information that were presented to Reiki students in the West, the practice of Reiki has stood the test of time. Today, Hawayo Takata is greatly respected within the Reiki community for the role she played in the growth of Reiki.

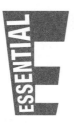

Were it not for Hawayo Takata's determination to assure that her students honored Reiki, it might never have spread as quickly or as far as it has. The secrecy on which she insisted and the costly fees she attached to taking Reiki classes made the attainment of the various Reiki levels extremely prestigious.

Reiki is a timeless healing energy. Its history has some interesting twists and turns, and parts of the story have yet to unravel. The fluidity of Reiki flows freely through our past, present, and future. When we attempt to restrict Reiki, it refuses to comply. Reiki practitioners and Reiki Masters have multiplied rapidly. Reiki is a gift bestowed on each person it visits. And each person who has opened up to Reiki offers his or her personal gift to the evolution of Reiki.

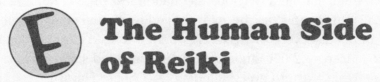

Chapter 18

The Human Side of Reiki

The cast of characters in the story of Reiki includes Reiki founder Dr. Mikao Usui, Dr. Chujiro Hayashi, and Mrs. Hawayo Takata. These figures are well known in the Reiki community. However, there are many more people who have followed in their footsteps and have made their own remarkable imprints in the sand, further expanding the Reiki system. In this chapter, you will learn about some of these people and what roles they have played in introducing so many of us to Reiki.

Mikao Usui

Dr. Mikaomi Usui (August 15, 1865–March 9, 1926), also known as Mikao Usui, was a Japanese Zen Buddhist, a businessman, spiritualist, and scholar. He was a married man with two children, a son and a daughter. His wife's name was Sadako Suzuki.

Usui participated in a religious meditation fast on Mt. Kurama in March 1921. During this fast he experienced a spiritual enlightenment that resulted in his discovery of Reiki. He opened a Reiki clinic in Japan and taught Reiki to over 2,000 students. Dr. Usui initiated sixteen individuals to Shinpiden, Reiki Master Level, including Dr. Chujiro Hayashi.

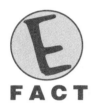

FACT

The Reiki organization Usui established was called Usui Reiki Ryoho Gakkai (*gakkai* is a Japanese word for "society"). Members of the society studied Reiki and held weekly meetings.

Presidents of Usui Reiki Ryoho Gakkai

Following Usui's death in 1926, Mr. Juzaburo Ushida became president of the Usui Reiki Ryoho Gakkai. It was Ushida who arranged the erection of Usui's memorial stone located at Usui's gravesite at the Saihoji Temple Cemetery in Tokyo, Japan. It was also Ushida who wrote the inscription that was carved on the stone.

Following Ushida's leadership in the Usui Reiki Ryoho Gakkai, the following Reiki Masters served as presidents:

1. Mr. Kanichi Taketomi
2. Mr. Yoshiharu Watanabe
3. Mr. Hoichi Wanami
4. Ms. Kimiko Koyama
5. Mr. Masayoshi Kondo

Chujiro Hayashi

Dr. Chujiro Hayashi (1879–May 10, 1940), noted today for organizing the basic hand placements used in Reiki, was originally a reservist in the

Japanese Imperial Navy. In 1925 Usui initiated him into Shinpiden, Reiki Master Level. In Takata's Reiki stories, she described a time when Hayashi became intrigued with Usui, who carried a burning torch in the daylight hours in order to draw attention to himself as a Reiki teacher. Supposedly, these two men met for the first time on just such an occasion.

It has since been documented that Hayashi was just one person among many navy personnel who showed interest in Reiki. Sometime after Dr. Usui's death in 1926, Hayashi broke away from the Usui Reiki Ryoho Gakkai and began to develop his own modified form of Reiki, eventually opening his own Reiki Ryoho clinic in Tokyo. Since his teaching clinic became well known among the affluent people of Japan, Hayashi's social status quickly rose to a level of great prominence in Tokyo.

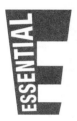

Before his death in 1940, Dr. Chujiro Hayashi initiated somewhere between thirteen and sixteen teachers to Shinpiden, Reiki Master Level. Two of the initiates were women, his wife, Chie Hayashi, and the Japanese-American Hawayo Takata.

Hawayo Takata

Mrs. Hawayo Takata (December 24, 1900–December 11, 1980) was born Hawayo Kawamuru on Christmas Eve on the island of Kauai, Hawaii. Her parents, Mr. and Mrs. Otogoro Kawamuru, named their daughter after the Hawaiian Islands.

Hawayo's father worked in the sugarcane fields. At age twelve Hawayo joined him to labor in the fields for one harvest season, but she had difficulty because she was small for her age. When she was older, she worked as a waitress and dishwasher at a soda fountain. Later, she spent several years employed as a housekeeper by a wealthy plantation owner. In time, she married the plantation's bookkeeper, Saichi Takata, and had two daughters with him. After Saichi died in October 1930 at the age of thirty-four, Takata continued on her own, working hard to provide for her two young daughters.

Takata suffered from severe abdominal pain due to a tumor, gallstones, and appendicitis. While visiting Japan she sought out medical care at a hospital in Tokyo. As she was being prepared for surgery, she heard a faint voice telling her that surgery was not needed, that there was another way. She asked the surgeon if there was an alternative treatment available. It was at this time that Takata became acquainted with Dr. Chujiro Hayashi at his Reiki clinic in Tokyo. Soon afterward, she began to receive daily treatments for her illness at the clinic. Hayashi agreed to empower Takata with four initiations that activated her to "Shoden," Reiki Level I, so she could do self-treatments.

After a few months, Dr. and Mrs. Hayashi invited Takata to stay at their home while she trained to be a Reiki practitioner. For the following year she worked mornings in the clinic and made house calls in the afternoon. When it was time for her to return to Hawaii in 1937, she received "Okuden," Reiki Level II empowerment from Hayashi. Dr. Hayashi and his daughter visited Takata in Hawaii to help her establish Reiki in Honolulu. Hayashi initiated Takata to "Shinpiden" in 1938 while visiting her in Hawaii, shortly before he returned home to Japan.

While continuing to teach Reiki in Hawaii, Takata also taught classes in the continental United States and in Canada in the 1970s. Her name for the system of Reiki that she taught was "the Usui System of Natural Healing" or "Usui Shiki Ryoho."

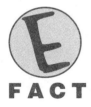

FACT

In 1976, Hawayo Takata trained her first four Master students, Virginia Samdahl, Barbara McCullough, Ethel Lombardi, and John Harvey Gray. Before her death in 1980, she trained and initiated twenty-two students as Reiki Masters.

Mrs. Takata's Twenty-Two Initiates

The names of the twenty-two Masters attuned by Hawayo Takata are widely publicized. Where are these people now and what is their involvement with Reiki? The brief information on the current status of these individuals that appears here was obtained courtesy of Usui Reiki Master Fran Brown's Web site, at ✍ *http://reikifranbrown.com.*

The Twenty-Two Initiates

Name	Status
George Araki	No longer teaches
Dorothy Baba	Deceased
Ursula Baylow	No longer teaches
Rick Bockner	Teaches Usui Reiki
Patricia Bowling Ewing	Teaches nontraditional Reiki
Barbara Brown	Deceased
Fran Brown	Teaches Usui Reiki
Phyllis Lei Furumoto	Teaches Usui Reiki
Beth Gray	No longer teaches
John Harvey Gray	Teaches Usui Reiki
Iris Ishikuro	Deceased
Harry Kuboi	Teaches nontraditional Reiki
Ethel Lombardi	Teaches nontraditional Reiki
Barbara McCullough	Teaches nontraditional Reiki
Mary McFadyen	Teaches Usui Reiki
Paul Mitchell	Teaches Usui Reiki
Bethel Phaigh	Deceased
Barbara Weber Ray	Teaches nontraditional Reiki, Radiance Technique
Shinobu Saito	Teaches Usui Reiki
Virginia Samdahl	Deceased
Wanja Twan	Teaches Usui Reiki
Kay Yamashita	Deceased

Additional information on Takata's twenty-two Masters has been researched and documented by Robert Fueston. Fueston received Usui Shiki Ryoho training from John Harvey Gray and Lourdes Gray. He maintains a frequently updated Web site at ✍ *www.reikisystem.com.*

George Araki

Araki received his doctorate in biological sciences from Stanford University for his work in ecological physiology. He became the director of the Center for Interdisciplinary Sciences and founded the Institute for Holistic Healing Studies (IHHS) in 1976. Araki was initiated into Reiki Master Level in 1979.

Rick Bockner

Bockner is a member of the Reiki Alliance. He received Reiki Level I on October 10, 1979; Reiki Level II on October 20, 1979; and his Reiki Master/Teacher Level degree on October 12, 1980.

Barbara Brown

Takata initiated Brown into the Reiki Master Level in October 1979 in Cherryville, Canada. Barbara Brown passed away on Easter Sunday, April 23, 2000.

Fran Brown

Fran Brown was the seventh Reiki Master initiated by Takata. She obtained her Reiki Level I on June 3, 1973, from Hawayo Takata. She received her Reiki Level II attunement from John Harvey Gray in 1976. On January 11, 1979, her Reiki Level II training was confirmed by Hawayo Takata and, soon after, she received her Master/Teacher Level training on January 15, 1979, in Keosauqua, Iowa. She is a member of the Reiki Alliance and has published a book entitled *Living Reiki: Takata's Teachings*.

Phyllis Lei Furumoto

Furumoto is the granddaughter of Hawayo Takata. She obtained her Reiki Master Level initiation in April 1979, in Keosauqua, Iowa. In 1983, the members of the Reiki Alliance designated her as the Grand Master and successor to her grandmother.

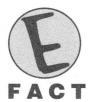

FACT

Among Takata's twenty-two Masters were three of her relatives, sister Kay Yamashita, cousin Iris Ishikuro, and granddaughter Phyllis Lei Furumoto. In some older Reiki texts, Shinobu Saito was mistakenly identified as Takata's cousin.

Beth Gray

Gray was initiated by John Harvey Gray, to whom she was married for a time. Later, in October of 1979, she received Master Level initiation from Hawayo Takata. Beth Gray is recognized for bringing Reiki to Australia and founding the largest full-time healing center in the United States. In the early 1990s she suffered a stroke and is now living in a care facility.

John Harvey Gray

John Harvey Gray was initiated into his Reiki Master Level on October 6, 1976, in Woodside, California. He was the third student Takata initiated as a Master. Gray is the founder and a minister of the Church of the Loving Servant, a nondenominational church devoted to spiritual healing. Gray has taught over 700 Reiki classes and initiated his current wife, Lourdes, as a Reiki Master/Teacher.

Iris Ishikuro

Hawayo Takata's cousin Iris Ishikuro was the tenth Master initiated by Takata. Ishikuro trained two people at Reiki Master Level—her daughter and Arthur Robertson.

Harry Kuboi

Kuboi was the sixth Reiki Master initiated by Hawayo Takata. He took his Reiki Level I training in 1974 and was initiated into the Reiki Master Level in April 1977. He has written two books on Reiki, *All of Reiki: Book One* and *All of Reiki: Book Two*.

Mary Alexandra McFadyen

McFadyen took her Reiki Level II training with John Harvey Gray and her Reiki Master Level training with Hawayo Takata. McFadyen founded Reiki Outreach International in 1990. She has recently published a Reiki book in German and is negotiating for an English-language version.

Paul Mitchell

Mitchell received his Reiki Master Level initiation in November 1979, in San Francisco, California. He is a member of the Reiki Alliance. Mitchell and Phyllis Lei Furumoto share a Web site, ✑*www.usuireiki.com.*

Mitchell had a Catholic upbringing and earned a philosophy degree at the University of San Francisco. He is the author of the student manual, *The Usui System of Natural Healing*, which is currently published in nine languages.

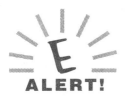

ALERT!

Perhaps because of its Japanese origin and unusual pronunciation, the word *Reiki* is commonly misspelled. Most frequent misspellings include "Reike," "Raykey," and "Rieki."

Bethel Phaigh

Bethel Phaigh was interested in alternative therapies and was introduced to Hawayo Takata by Barbara Brown. She was initiated to Master Level in the late 1970s. Phaigh was the author of two books: *Gestalt and the Wisdom of the Kahunas* and *Journey into Consciousness*. The second book is an autobiography of her life, and it was never published. Phaigh died on January 3, 1986.

Barbara Weber Ray

Dr. Barbara Weber Ray received her Reiki Level I initiation on August 20, 1978; her Reiki Level II on October 2, 1978; and her Master Level on September 1, 1979. She holds a Ph.D. in the humanities.

Ray developed the Radiance Technique with its seven levels of Reiki training, which she claims was taught to her by Hawayo Takata before her death in 1980. She founded the Radiance Technique International Association, Inc., previously known as the American Reiki Association, Inc. Barbara Weber Ray has also authored several books, including *The 'Reiki' Factor in The Radiance Technique* and *The Authentic Reiki*.

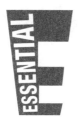

After Takata's death, two of her twenty-two Masters, Phyllis Lei Furumoto and Barbara Weber Ray, each claimed to have been named as Takata's successor. This created a rift in the Reiki community in the West. However, it has since become standard protocol for Reiki Masters to instruct their students to honor and respect all Reiki paths, no matter what system they teach.

Shinobu Saito

Saito received her Reiki Level I in 1976, her Level II in 1978, and her Reiki Master Level in May 1980 in Palo Alto, California. She continues to teach Usui Reiki today and has trained some Masters in Japan.

Virginia Samdahl

Samdahl was the first of Takata's students to receive Master Level. She was initiated to Reiki Level I in 1974, Reiki Level II in 1975, and Master Level in 1976. Barbara Derrick Lugenbeel published a biography of Virginia Samdahl, titled *Virginia Samdahl: Reiki Master Healer* (the biography is currently out of print). Samdahl passed away on March 4, 1994.

Wanja Twan

Twan received her Master Level initiation in 1979 in Cherryville, Canada. She is a member of the Reiki Alliance and author of *In the Light of a Distant Star: A Spiritual Journey Bringing the Unseen into the Seen*. Twan taught Reiki in Russia and Sweden.

Reiki Historians

Thanks to a handful of Reiki Masters who were not content to accept Takata's Reiki stories at face value without first researching their validity, the true facts are now emerging. Trips have been made to Japan to research the lives of Dr. Usui, Dr. Hayashi, and the dawn of Reiki. The whole story has yet to be completely disclosed, and indeed may never be fully known, but, as each piece of the puzzle is found, we will get closer to assembling the whole picture. Listed here are a few Reiki Masters with the requisite detective skills whom we can thank for their diligence and perseverance in researching Reiki's historical roots:

- Hiroshi Doi
- Dave King
- Frank Arjava Petter
- William Lee Rand
- Melissa Riggall
- Diane Stein

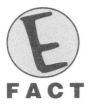

FACT

Mieko Mitsui has been credited for reintroducing Reiki to Japan in 1984. She is a student of Barbara Weber Ray's Radiance Technique. Mitsui was authorized to teach only Levels I and II in Japan. Mitsui attuned Hiroshi Doi to Levels I and II prior to his membership in Usui Reiki Ryoho Gakkai.

Hiroshi Doi

Doi became a member of Japan's Usui Reiki Ryoho Gakkai in October 1993. The sixth president of the Gakkai, Kimiko Koyama, initiated Doi. Through his association with the Usui Reiki Ryoho Gakkai, he came to learn the differences between the modified Reiki as taught by Hawayo Takata and the traditional Japanese Reiki. Doi established Gendai Reiki-ho (the Modern Reiki Healing Method), which is a combination of the Eastern and Western traditions.

Dave King and Melissa Riggall

Dave King and Melissa Riggall learned Usui Reiki from Usui-sensei
(Usui teacher) Yuji Onuki while vacationing in Morocco in 1971. In 1995
King and Riggall attained Usui-Do Shichidan (the seventh level of Usui-Do,
the original name of traditional Japanese Reiki) in Japan from Tatsumi-
sensei. King and Riggall worked together to translate various documents
from copies of Tatsumi's notes, comparing them to notes Riggall obtained
from their Usui Reiki training with Onuki.

Dave King also made frequent trips to Japan, as well as to other
countries, to better understand Usui's teachings. King now teaches Usui-
Do. He lives in Toronto, Canada, with his wife, Pat. Riggall died in the
Heilongjiang province of China on March 12, 2003.

Frank Arjava Petter

Petter is recognized for returning Reiki to its homeland. He was the
first Westerner to teach Reiki Master/Teacher Level in Japan. Petter is the
author of *Reiki Fire; Reiki: The Legacy of Dr. Usui;* and *The Original
Reiki Handbook of Dr. Mikao Usui*, and he coauthored *The Spirit of
Reiki* along with William Lee Rand and Walter Lübeck. These works detail
his research into Japanese Reiki history. Petter currently lives in Germany.

William Lee Rand

Rand is founder of the International Center for Reiki Training. He is a
Master/Teacher of Usui and Karuna Reiki. He has authored *Reiki: The
Healing Touch* and *Reiki for a New Millennium,* as well as several other
Reiki publications. Rand is also the publisher of *Reiki News.* He received
his first Reiki training from Bethel Phaigh in 1981. Rand received Reiki
Level I in 1981, Reiki Level II in 1982, and became a Reiki Master/Teacher
in 1989. He has since studied with many other Reiki Masters.

Diane Stein

Diane Stein is a prominent figure in the Women's Spirituality Movement.
Stein became a Reiki Master/Teacher in 1990 and now teaches

nontraditional Reiki. In 1995, she published *Essential Reiki: A Complete Guide to an Ancient Healing Art.* Through this controversial book, Stein defied the tradition of keeping Reiki shrouded in secrecy by publishing Reiki's sacred symbols and describing the attunement process. *Essential Reiki* opened the eyes of many to the possibility that the true Reiki story had yet to be told, making some people uncomfortable, and others hopeful.

Modern-Day Reiki Pioneers

The Reiki revolution has virtually exploded. Many paths abound, each with its own twists and turns. The Internet has played a gigantic role in spreading Reiki. At the time of this writing, a Google.com keyword search for "Reiki" brings up over a million links. Light and Adonea and Vincent Amador maintain megasize Reiki Web sites with loads of useful information (see Appendix C for these, and other, Web site addresses).

Light and Adonea

Light and Adonea, teachers of the Usui Reiki Ryoho tradition, founded the Southwestern Usui Reiki Association. They have also been trained in other Reiki traditions—Gendai Reiki-ho Shihan, Usui Tera-Mai, Brahma Satya Reiki, Radiance Technique, and Karuna Reiki. Together, they have written several Reiki manuals and trained hundreds of Reiki students.

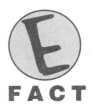

FACT

Well-known for their growing interactive Web site featuring an Internet directory on Usui Sensei's Original System of Reiki, Light and Adonea have been serving the Internet community since 1997.

Vincent Amador

Amador's Web site, Living Reiki, Being Reiki, and his e-books (*Reiki Plain and Simple* and *Reiki Ryoho Plain and Simple)* are jam-packed with information and perceptions on the subject of Reiki. Amador doesn't shy away from expressing his opinions on what Reiki should and shouldn't be.

Reiki Lineages

"What is your Reiki lineage?" This question, occasionally posed to Reiki practitioners, seems to suggest that some teachers might be better qualified to teach Reiki. But a person's Reiki lineage is merely the progression of Master/student relationships that is traced back, in one way or another, to Hawayo Takata. It is not at all an indicator of how pure or powerful a person's teaching strengths or abilities may be.

If a particular lineage is important to the student, by all means, the student should procure a teacher who can verify that desired lineage. But, it would be hoped that other factors would also be considered in evaluating a person's knowledge of and familiarity with Reiki.

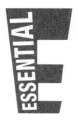

Reiki teachers attract students who can learn from them, but Reiki students may also have something to teach their Masters. Don't allow lineage, or lack of lineage, to get in the way of learning Reiki from the most appropriate teacher.

The human side of Reiki will always be reflected through the histories of those people who practice Reiki and allow it to play a major role in how they live their lives. Whether or not Usui literally carried a lighted torch to draw crowds of people to learn about Reiki, his teachings have won a multitude of followers. From among these followers many variations of the Reiki systems have emerged. (E)

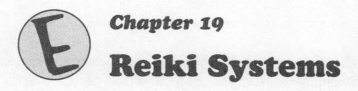

Chapter 19
Reiki Systems

Many variations of Reiki have been developed since Dr. Usui first made his discovery, and new versions of Reiki continue to evolve today. Each system offers its own unique twist to the simple art of Reiki. Some of the variant Reiki systems imply mysterious or metaphysical origins. Several of these methodologies claim to have made use of newly created or rediscovered traditional Reiki systems that are somehow superior to the original documented teachings.

A Variety of Systems

Once Hawayo Takata introduced Reiki to the West, her established tradition of passing down information about Reiki from teacher to student through spoken word, rather than written text, allowed leeway for modifications through interpretational differences. The history of Reiki took on different flavorings, depending on how each teacher retold the stories to help students better understand and remember the teachings.

The Reiki kanji symbols used in passing attunements and distance healing were written down on paper only for a brief time during instruction in order to facilitate memorization during instruction. After memorization, the papers were destroyed to keep the symbols secret. Relying on memory alone to preserve the teachings of Reiki left plenty of room for mistakes to enter in and for blatant deviations from the original materials to become incorporated into the works.

Reiki Masters Break into Two Camps

A major split occurred among the twenty-two Masters initiated by Hawayo Takata after her death, when two individuals declared themselves to be Hawayo Takata's successor. Phyllis Lei Furumoto, granddaughter of Hawayo Takata, proclaimed she was the lineage bearer and Grand Master of Reiki. In 1983, Furumoto helped to organize the Reiki Alliance.

For her part, Barbara Weber Ray claims to be the successor of Holders of The Intact Master Keys of Reiki. In 1980, Ray founded the American Reiki Association, Inc., which was later renamed the Radiance Technique International Association, Inc.

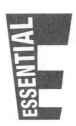

In addition to this split, many other students branched out from the original teaching and developed their own systems of practicing and teaching Reiki. These systems are covered in this chapter.

The Original Systems

Dr. Mikao Usui is internationally recognized as the founder of Reiki. His findings and experiences of using Universal Life Energy for healing were passed down to others. Usui's teachings remain the foundation of most of the Reiki systems that are in use today.

Usui Reiki Ryoho, as it originated from Mikao Usui, is still practiced in Japan. It teaches spiritual development and self-healing through empowerments and meditations. These empowerments, such as Reiju, are used instead of the attunements in order to open and clear the Reiki passageways within the initiates.

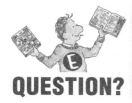

QUESTION?

What is Reiju?
Reiju is the empowerment process used by Usui to pass Reiki to his students. It is the direct result of the spiritual enlightenment that Usui received during his meditation fast on Mt. Kurama in March 1921.

Usui Shiki Ryoho

The Usui Shiki Ryoho system emerged from the Usui-Hayashi lineage. This is the traditional Usui System of Natural Healing that made its way to the United States from Japan through the teachings of Mrs. Hawayo Takata. The primary principles taught in this book are based on the fundamental teachings of this system, its principles, attunements, symbols, and hand placements.

Raku Kai Reiki

Arthur Robertson developed Raku Kai Reiki. He designed this system to enhance the Reiki experience. Arthur Robertson's lineage is Mikao Usui–Churjiro Hayashi–Hawayo Takata–Iris Ishikuro.

Raku Kai Reiki was a precursor to Usui/Tibetan Reiki, Vajra Reiki, Karuna Reiki, and Tera-Mai Reiki. Raku Kai incorporates the Hui Yin, the Breath of the Fire Dragon, Kundalini breathing, and other Tibetan practices/symbolism.

Usui/Tibetan Reiki

Usui/Tibetan Reiki combines Usui Shiki Ryoho Reiki, Raku Kai Reiki, and Advanced Reiki Training (ART). This system, popularized by William Lee Rand and Diane Stein, has four levels of training: Reiki I, II, IIIa, and III/Master. Level IIIa of this system, also referred to as ART, consists of a variety of add-on techniques such as the use of crystal grids, guides, healing attunement, psychic surgery, meditations, and Tibetan symbols.

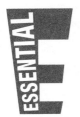

A lot of the Reiki systems and names are trademarked. The owner of a trademark has the exclusive right to use it on the product, and any related products, that it was intended to identify.

Trademarked Systems

In 1997, Phyllis Lei Furumoto attempted to trademark the word *Reiki*, along with the terms *Usui Shiki Ryoho* and *Usui System*. Her attempts failed. However, specialized Reiki systems, such as Tera-Mai and Karuna Reiki, have successfully been trademarked, as their inceptions were sufficiently documented to satisfy trademark standards.

Authentic Reiki

Authentic Reiki, Real Reiki, and The Radiance Technique are registered service marks of The Radiance Technique International Association, Inc. Dr. Barbara Weber Ray, one of Hawayo Takata's twenty-two Masters, claims that Mrs. Takata instructed her in the seven degrees of the Usui System of Natural Healing and passed the complete Usui Reiki Keys to her before Takata's death in 1980.

Tera-Mai Reiki and Seichem

Tera-Mai Reiki combines Usui Reiki and Seichem. Seichem (pronounced SAY-keem) is an Egyptian energy-based healing system. Its name was derived from the Egyptian word *sekhem,* which means "power" or "energy." *Sekhem,* in Seichem healing, is equivalent to ki in Reiki healing.

Together, Reiki and Seichem represent the four elements: Reiki (earth), joined with the three Seichem elements, sakara (fire), sophi-el (water), and angelic light (air/ether). There are various ways of giving treatment using the four different elemental healing rays—earth, water, fire, and wind.

Tera-Mai Trademark Information

Tera-Mai is the registered trademark of Kathleen Milner (USA), author of *Reiki & Other Rays of Touch Healing*. Kathleen was originally trained in traditional Reiki and Seichem. Later, she was "led by Spirit" to use an updated attunement process and symbols, and this is how the Tera-Mai Reiki was created. In 1995 the Tera-Mai trademark was set up to protect and maintain the integrity of these new attunements. Under the terms of the trademark, Tera-Mai Masters are not permitted to perform attunements from any other Reiki or Seichem system. This assures that all attunees receive the same initiations, no matter who the teacher is. All registered Tera-Mai Masters are required to adapt to any additional changes in the Tera-Mai system as they are "brought in from Spirit" via Kathleen Milner.

Karuna Reiki

Karuna Reiki is the registered trademark of the International Center for Reiki Training. William Lee Rand, founder and director of the International Center for Reiki Training, worked with some of his Reiki students to develop Karuna Reiki. Rand and his students experimented with symbols gathered from Reiki Masters with whom Rand had collaborated in his earlier travels while teaching and practicing Reiki.

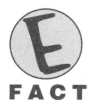

Karuna Reiki, also defined as Reiki of Compassion, was trade-marked in 1995 by the International Center for Reiki Training. Karuna, a Sanskrit word, is used in both Hinduism and Buddhism to signify "compassionate action."

Karuna Reiki classes offer two levels, two attunements, four Master symbols, and eight treatment symbols. Rand emphasizes that he did not create the Karuna Reiki symbols. He agrees that Karuna Reiki employs some of the same symbols used by other schools and systems, but he also claims that the attunement process and intention in Karuna Reiki are different. During a Karuna Reiki treatment, the practitioner chants and intones the names of these symbols. Prior Reiki Master training is a prerequisite to taking Karuna Reiki.

Lightarian Reiki

Lightarian Reiki was introduced in 1997 through the channeling efforts of Jeannine Marie Jelm, cofounder of the Lightarian Institute for Global Human Transformation located in Sedona, Arizona. Jelm is a spiritual counselor and conscious channel for the Ascended Masters.

Jelm claims that Lightarian Reiki is based on information revealed to her by Ascended Master Buddha. The intent of Lightarian Reiki is to awaken humanity to six higher vibrational bands of Reiki energies. Via Jelm's channeling, it has been suggested that Lightarian Reiki occupies the six highest bands of a total of eight vibrational bands within the Reiki spectrum. No symbols are used in the Lightarian Reiki system of Reiki. Lightarian Reiki consists of four levels of attunements: Levels I and II; III; IV; and V and VI.

Lightarian Attunements Level I and II

The initial Lightarian attunements for Level I and II are achieved through a guided meditation. They serve as an introduction to the energies of Ascended Master Buddha and offer the primary Lightarian Reiki Principles. This guided meditation can be experienced in person, over the telephone, through e-mail, or remotely.

Lightarian Attunement Level III

The third attunement is an introduction to Gaea, the Earth Mother. Gaea's energies provide the attunee with help in his or her grounding and advancement of personal self-healing.

Lightarian Attunement Level IV

The fourth attunement connects the attunee to the vibrational healing energies of the God Source.

Lightarian Attunement Levels V and VI

This final attunement joins Ascended Master Sanada (called Jesus here on Earth) together with Gaea, the God Source, and Ascended Master Buddha. This union of healing energies creates a visualization tool, called the Divine Healing Chamber, which can be utilized to bring about extraordinary healing results.

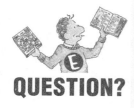

QUESTION?

Who are the Ascended Masters?
Ascended Masters are enlightened spiritual beings who once lived on earth. Over the course of many lifetimes, they managed to complete all of their spiritual lessons and have ascended back to their divine source. They offer spiritual advice and compassion to those of us who are still in the physical realm by staying in spirit communication with chosen souls that are currently incarnate.

Transformational Reiki

Transformational Reiki is taught as the first level of Reiki Mystery School, a two-day class taught by Karyn and Steve Mitchell. Steve and Karyn are teachers of the Usui Shiki Ryoho School of Reiki as well as instructors and members of the Midwest International University for the Healing Arts.

Transformational Reiki introduces serious Reiki students to the Interdimensional Chakra System and the Interdimensional Bodies that lead them beyond the structure and limitations of the physical body. Students are taught about a healing field (the Unisonium) where two people (the healer and the person being healed) meet and create a more intense energy potential for healing. This ancient Tibetan attunement links the soul to Interdimensional Reality and the soul's purpose. Meditations taught include the following:

- Meeting your Interdimensional Guide
- Interdimensional chakras, their energy, planes of existence, and potential
- Soul's purpose
- Melting into the Unisonium

Wei Chi Tibetan Reiki

This system of Reiki is publicized as having been "rediscovered" through channeled information received by Kevin Ross Emery. The channeled entity, Wei Chi, claims that he is a 5,000-year-old Tibetan monk. Along with his brothers, Wei Chi was a creator of the original Reiki system. Wei Chi asserts that much of the original teachings have been lost through the centuries.

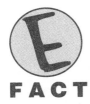

FACT

Tommy Hensel and Kevin Ross Emery, promoters of Wei Chi Tibetan Reiki, have called Wei Chi Tibetan Reiki a Therapeutic Reiki and describe it as less passive than the relaxation and stress-reduction actions of traditional Reiki as most people understand it.

In this new system, the recipient and the practitioner hold dialogue before, during, and after the treatment. The practitioner not only channels Reiki's ki energies, but intuitively gleans information from the recipient as well. This information is shared with the recipient as a means to help him or her become a more active player, empowering the recipient to heal more deeply.

Either a third person takes notes or a tape recorder is used to record any information that is communicated during the session. There are no sequenced hand placements in Wei Chi Tibetan Reiki. The practitioner intuitively moves his or her hands wherever they are drawn. After the session, the practitioner and recipient discuss how it went, laying out a plan for the recipient to undertake in order to continue the healing process.

The treatment of Wei Chi Tibetan Reiki can only be performed if the recipient meets the following two conditions:

1. The recipient has to acknowledge that she is responsible for everything that happens in her life, for both good and bad, and that all life experiences teach us important lessons.

2. The recipient has to be willing to participate in her own healing.

If the recipient does not meet these requirements, the Wei Chi practitioner will refuse to treat her.

More Variations

As a result of individuals adding other healing modalities to Reiki systems already in place, the following offshoot systems have been developed as well. The inventors of these systems are really nothing more than bakers adding ingredients to spice up a cake recipe that is already sufficiently palatable. As we strive to reinvent the wheel, it is important to remember that the wheel spins effectively without any fancy bells and whistles attached to it. To fully benefit from Reiki, it is not productive to become overly absorbed in intellectual studies of the many convoluted concepts. Experiencing Reiki in its simplest form is enough.

Gendai Reiki-ho

Sensei Hiroshi Doi founded Gendai Reiki-ho. It is primarily a Japanese style of Reiki. Translated into English, *Gendai Reiki-ho* means "Modern Reiki Method for Healing."

However, Gendai Reiki-ho also includes influences from Western Reiki systems and other healing modalities, as well as influences from the Western Reiki systems founded by Sensei Hiroshi Doi. In his teachings, Doi explains to his students the differences in the system, clarifying what material is "traditional Japanese Reiki" and what is "Western Reiki." There are four levels of teachings in Gendai Reiki-ho: Shoden, Okuden, Shinpiden, and Gokuikaiden.

Karuna Ki

Vincent P. Amador developed the Karuna Ki system, also called the Way of Compassionate Energy. In no way associated with Karuna Reiki, this system is a culmination of "healing art" and "meditative practices." Amador has chosen to keep this system free of limiting trademarks, allowing teachers to add information to its basic teachings, as they feel inclined.

Kundalini Reiki

Kundalini Reiki is an easy-to-use healing technique that requires no intense study or complex procedures. Its attunement process allows the chakras to be opened wider to allow Kundalini energy to flow more easily and fully through your body.

Kundalini Reiki was introduced by a native of Denmark, Mr. Ole Gabrielsen, known best for his bestselling meditation CDs.

Kundalini Reiki is a direct result of Mr. Gabrielsen's communications with Ascended Master Kuthumi. Mahatma Kuthumi lived in the early nineteenth century. He was born to a Punjabi family that settled in Kashmir. Records indicate that he attended Oxford University in 1850 and is believed to have contributed "The Dream of Ravan" to *The Dublin University Magazine* around 1854. His final years were lived in seclusion in Shigatse, Tibet. Letters that he had sent to his students from Tibet are now on file with the British Museum.

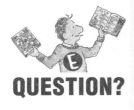

QUESTION?

What is Kundalini energy?
The Kundalini energy, also referred to as Kundalini fire, is a channel of energy that flows upward from the root chakra (located near the coccyx) to the crown chakra (located on the top of the head). Having an open Kundalini indicates that there has been a complete cleansing of the chakras and that the body parts and the energy channels are unblocked.

Kundalini Reiki Level I

There are three Kundalini Reiki attunements. The first attunement opens the Reiki channel and also prepares the attunee for Level II. The crown, heart, and hand chakras are opened and strengthened. At this stage, the attunee learns how to give a complete healing treatment and how to heal remotely.

Kundalini Reiki Level II

The second attunement is called the Kundalini Awakening. The main energy channel opens gently and the Kundalini fire is lit. The flame of the Kundalini reaches upward to the solar plexus chakra in preparation for the complete Kundalini rising that takes place in Level III. A specific meditation is taught that increases the power of the Kundalini and cleanses the chakra system,

Kundalini Reiki Level III

The third attunement is the Master Level of Kundalini Reiki. The attunee's throat, solar plexus, hara, and root chakras are opened. The previous attunements are strengthened as well. A full rising of the Kundalini takes place during this attunement. The student learns how to attune crystals and other objects to serve as Reiki channels, and he or she is taught how to pass attunements for all levels of Kundalini Reiki.

Tummo Rei Ki

Another Reiki system involving the awakening of the Kundalini is called Tummo Rei Ki. This system is said to be very different from other Usui-based Reiki traditions and was supposedly taught by Buddha as a means to achieve enlightenment in the scope of one lifetime.

Shamballa Reiki

John Armitage developed the Shamballa Multidimensional Healing System. Shamballa is promoted as not only a system of healing, but also as a way of accelerating your spiritual development. Classes are available from Level I through Master/Teacher Level. The full system includes 352 symbols, the DNA symbol, Mahatma initiation, and encompasses a twelve-chakra system.

A high priest at the Temple of Healing who resided in the ancient civilization of Atlantis is credited as the originator of Shamballa Reiki. This high priest, now known as Ascended Master St. Germain, went into the far mountains away from the central temples of Atlantis, creating his own separate tribe of Atlanteans called the Inspirers. In that lifetime, St. Germain was given twenty-two symbols.

When Atlantis was destroyed, St. Germain journeyed with several of his people, the Inspirers, to ancient Tibet. St. Germain and the Inspirers chose not to give the full twenty-two symbols to any individuals in that region in order to protect Reiki from possible corruption. Shamballa practitioners feel that the Reiki system, as it is practiced today, is an incomplete system. It was revealed to Dr. John Armitage by the Collective Consciousness of the Lords and Ladies of Shamballa (the Ascended Masters) that there are 352 symbols in the Shamballa Reiki System, which correspond to 352 levels, or initiations.

Rainbow Reiki

Rainbow Reiki is a spiritual way developed by Walter Lübeck as a result of his in-depth research into the many healing modalities, including Usui Reiki, shamanism, feng shui, meditation, human psychology, holistic communication sciences, and healing body. The three pillars of Rainbow Reiki are love, self-responsibility, and consciousness.

Violet Flame Reiki

Violet Flame Reiki is a newly discovered form of Reiki dedicated to Lady Quan Yin, the goddess of compassion and mercy. One day, while Ivy Moore was meditating upon Quan Yin and wishing to develop better healing skills using Reiki, she channeled approximately forty symbols. The focus of this Reiki system is clearing away the ego and healing with a pure heart. Usui Reiki Level II and beyond are prerequisites for learning Violet Flame Reiki.

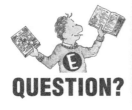

QUESTION?

Who is Lady Quan Yin?
Lady Quan Yin is one of the deities in the Buddhist tradition. She is best known as the goddess of mercy. Quan Yin's role as Buddhist Madonna is comparable to that of Mary, the mother of Jesus, in Christianity.

From a Common Source

Reiki is pure in its essence. However, the vibrational energies of Reiki, while being channeled through our bodies, blend in with our individual vibrational identities. This means that, for each of us, our experiences with Reiki can be distinctly different. Different Reiki systems were ultimately derived from those varied experiences. Human nature has urged some people to challenge the past systems of Reiki and to pioneer new paths.

The roots of Reiki and the various Reiki systems that have developed since its inception are evidence that Reiki is and will continue to be an evolving energy healing modality. The absolute essence of Reiki is constant, but it will take on different forms, depending on the personality of the practitioner who uses it.

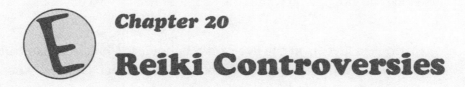

Chapter 20

Reiki Controversies

When someone begins to question the status quo, controversy usually rears its ugly face. Controversy is likely to crop up almost any time people discuss spirituality, religion, or ethics. Since Reiki is a healing art that has a spiritual vein but is not based on any one religion, there is much diversity among those who are drawn to it. Therefore, it is to be expected that Reiki controversies will sometimes arise among its followers.

Opposing Attitudes

Discussing opposing views will sometimes lead to strife and discord among family members, neighbors, and associates. Arguments are bound to occur when one person feels he or she knows the truth and decides that everyone else is ignorant or misinformed. However, attitudes of overt righteousness and superiority do not belong within the scope of Reiki's love energies.

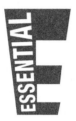

Truth, like love, is in the eye of the beholder. What feels like truth to one person may feel like deception to another. Our life experiences teach us what feels right and what feels wrong. However, it is never acceptable to impose one's perception of truth on another person. Each person must find his or her own truth.

Hidden Truths

Usui Reiki has a history of its teachings being cloaked in secrecy. Instructors told their students that the Reiki materials and procedures they were taught were to be kept confidential. It was emphasized that the sacredness of Reiki was too important to be divulged to outsiders.

Integrity is a common trait possessed by healers and all people who are drawn to Reiki. Reiki practitioners' integrity played a tremendous role in keeping Reiki a secret for a very long time. Practitioners wanted to honor promises they made to their Reiki Masters to keep the knowledge of Reiki private. There was even a large tuition fee of $10,000 attached to receiving mastership. This high price was intended to assure that only an elite few, those who were totally committed to and appreciative of Reiki, would have complete access to its mysteries.

Eventually, however, it was some practitioners' sense of personal integrity that led them to question why Reiki methodologies should be kept hidden. They also questioned why Reiki should be available only to those who could afford it. These practitioners wanted to be able to share Reiki's healing benefits with more people, and they decided that Reiki classes should be readily available to everyone. For these people, spreading Reiki was more important than honoring their promise to their Reiki instructor. Consequently, their Reiki class fees were reduced to more affordable prices,

Reiki training became more accessible to the masses, and controversy erupted soon after.

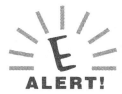

ALERT!

Make peace with your attitudes toward Reiki issues and never mind that your attitude might be offensive to others or in opposition to their feelings and beliefs. You're still a practitioner of Reiki, no matter which side of a controversial issue you choose to believe in.

Changing Attitudes

There is a positive side to controversy. Our attitudes and opinions are best kept flexible and open to change. When an argument is persuasive, you'll want to be able to switch gears without feeling too much resistance. It is helpful to re-evaluate your opinions from time to time to make sure that you are not bogged down with obsolete or regressive thinking processes.

Remember, Reiki is about balance. "Mule heads," people who are stubbornly resistant to change, and plain old "suckers," people who are too easily influenced by almost anything, are both going to meet in the middle as their energies balance when Reiki is routinely applied. With Reiki's overt influence, flexibility merges with rigidity. In other words, the adaptable vine will stiffen as it intertwines around the staff, and the rigid staff will bend to some degree while under the gentle wrap of the vine.

Agree to Disagree

Heated discussions among practitioners over Reiki controversies do eventually cool down. It is the Reiki way for practitioners to respect all paths chosen by other practitioners. It is not for us to accept or reject another practitioner's attitude. We can all agree to disagree and get along just fine.

Money Matters

When some Usui Reiki Masters broke away from the tradition of charging excessive prices for Reiki attunements and training, it was a bit of a blow to others who had established steady income from teaching Reiki students. They now had to contend with competitive pricing and, with more Masters being attuned, they would also have more teachers to compete with. It was a scary position for them to be placed in. Not only did they have concerns about their future incomes, but they were forced to question their beliefs regarding Reiki as well. Were they willing to reduce their prices in order to stay competitive with those who had broken rank? Or would they keep their promises to Mrs. Takata's teaching and continue to charge the prices she had put in place?

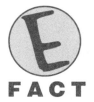

FACT

Mrs. Hawayo Takata set the price of $10,000 for Reiki Master/ Teacher Level training. In addition, for the next twelve months the newly attuned Reiki Master/Teacher was expected to turn over all Reiki class earnings to the Master who had initiated him or her.

Members of the Reiki Alliance remain in keeping with the class fees determined by Mrs. Takata. Today, Alliance members' fees for Reiki Level I is $150, Level II is $500, and Reiki Master Level is $10,000.

On the other hand, Usui Reiki Master/Teachers who are not Alliance members set their own prices. Average pricing for Reiki Level I is $75 to $150. Reiki Level II is $125 to $250, and Reiki Master Level is $500 to $2,000.

What Is a Fair Price to Pay?

When comparing the prices of different Reiki classes, some may assume that the higher-priced classes must offer greater value. Another assumption that follows in this same vein is that reduced Reiki class fees would equate to reduced value of training. While this may be true in some cases, it should not be taken as necessarily true for all. Value cannot always be measured in money. There are certainly Reiki students who graduated from higher-priced Reiki classes feeling terribly disappointed. On the other hand, there are some students who received free Reiki training from their teachers and were very pleased with the outcome.

The price charged for a Reiki class should meet the following conditions:

1. The teacher charges a certain amount of money that he or she believes is necessary in order to feel valued as a teacher.

2. The student pays the sum of money that he or she feels is fair and reasonable for the amount of training involved.

If both of these two conditions are not satisfied, the teacher or the student, or both, will feel shortchanged. Either the teacher will feel undervalued or the student will feel cheated.

Room for Negotiation

Reiki class fees are often negotiable. If you feel drawn to a particular instructor but are unwilling or unable to pay the fee that is advertised, it is certainly permissible to approach the instructor to see if an alternate arrangement might be possible. However, respect the teacher if he or she tells you that the class fee is not subject to change. And please don't try to "guilt" or "goad" a Reiki Master into reducing his or her fee. To do so would not make for a good start in building a healthy teacher/student relationship. The class fee is part of the teacher/student contract. If both parties cannot agree on a fee, the contract was simply not meant to be. Class fees aside, no Reiki teacher should ever feel obligated to accept a student. Also, no student should feel obligated to take a class from a particular teacher.

Energy Exchange

Charging fees for Reiki attunements and treatments is passionately debated among Reiki practitioners. Takata taught her students that there must always be an "energy exchange" in order for Reiki to be valued by the recipient. Takata held the position that anything received as charity would not be fully valued.

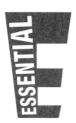

It has been argued that Reiki can be appreciated only when it is paid for in some way or if a sacrifice of some kind is made in exchange for it. Unfortunately, this reasoning does have a ring of truth to it for some people. Many people have conditioned themselves into believing that healing can only be gained through the exchange of money and labor.

The most common "energy exchange" offered in return for a Reiki treatment is money, but some practitioners are open to bartering. They will accept agreed-upon services or goods in place of money in return for a Reiki treatment.

Another controversy that has risen out of Takata's "energy exchange" notion is that it is in direct conflict with the fact that practitioners do not give away their own energy when conducting a treatment. If practitioners are merely serving as conduits for Reiki to flow through their bodies and they are not depleting their own energy, why should they require energy replenishment in the form of an exchange?

The argument goes like this: If Reiki is a universal energy, free to all, why should anyone have to pay for it? This reasoning makes sense, until you consider the time and efforts involved in conducting Reiki treatments. Once you do that, you'll realize that there is nothing wrong in practitioners expecting payment for their time and efforts.

In the end, whether to charge or not charge for giving Reiki attunements and treatments is entirely the practitioner's personal choice. A practitioner should not have to defend his or her reasoning for choosing to expect payment. As long as the price is agreed on before the treatment, both practitioner and recipient will be gratified.

The "True" Lineage Bearer

Lineage is what traces a Reiki practitioner's history, much like genealogy traces your bloodline and family roots. Your Reiki lineage denotes who your Reiki training originally came from, who that person received his training from, and so on down the line of Reiki Masters/Teachers. It is from these individuals' teachings and their shared experiences that Reiki will go to you, and, in turn, through your practice of Reiki, Reiki will continue to evolve and go to others.

Takata attuned twenty-two Masters. This means that there are twenty-two individuals whose lineage reads as follows: Usui–Hayashi–Takata. Although Takata claimed that she was the titled successor to Chujiro Hayashi, this was not true. Neither was Hayashi the titled successor to Usui. Now that it is known that Takata misrepresented her position, it seems a trivial matter that there are two of Takata's Masters in disagreement as to who should rightfully hold the title of Grand Master. On the one hand, Phyllis Lei Furumoto maintains that she is her grandmother's Spiritual Lineage Bearer; on the other hand, Barbara Weber Ray continues to declare herself as successor to Takata, claiming that she received additional information from Takata that no one else was made privy to, that is, the Seven Degrees of Reiki.

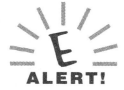
ALERT!

Because Reiki energies tend to put recipients in a state of relaxation, take precautions not to send long-distance Reiki treatments during time periods when the recipient will be operating a motor vehicle or performing any other type of function that requires him to be consciously awake and fully alert.

This division of Reiki teachings into two opposing camps has become significant in the history and evolution of Usui Reiki. The split between Furumoto and Ray in the Reiki community provoked questions in the minds of many practitioners, forcing them to evaluate what paths were right for them. The controversy that remains on this issue is only in the minds of some practitioners who have concluded that their chosen path is the only right one and that differing paths that others have chosen are wrong. Since this initial division of Reiki, further offshoots from basic Reiki teachings have occurred. Reiki has taken many paths and continues to branch out in many different directions.

Attunement Concerns

Reiki practitioners and the people who are just learning about Reiki frequently discuss the purposes behind the Reiki attunement ritual. Understandably, many people who are new to Reiki are both intrigued and confused by the attunement process.

Some people feel that Reiki attunements are mostly symbolic in nature and have little significance in regard to the actual application of Reiki treatments. These people recognize that ceremonies such as baptisms, weddings, and graduations represent milestones in a person's lifetime, and are not milestones *in themselves*. For them, the Reiki attunement rite represents their commitment to service. The Reiki student commits to administering her healing hands for self-healing and to assist in healing others.

On the other hand, spiritually oriented Reiki students tend to look upon attunements as mystical experiences that have meaning that goes beyond ceremony. They take the Reiki attunement ritual very seriously and believe that the attunement is a spiritually transforming experience that will forever change them. If Reiki students of this mindset end up feeling that they did not have a profound enough experience, they may worry that their attunement didn't "take" or that it was done improperly.

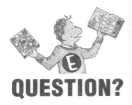

QUESTION?

What is a booster attunement?
A booster Reiki attunement is an optional attunement that can be given to anyone who has already been initiated as a Reiki practitioner. Its purpose, in general, is to "jump-start" or increase the flow of Reiki through the body.

Reiki Boosters

Some practitioners feel that repeated booster attunements give them more power and strengthen their ability to be clearer conduits. Others feel that booster attunements are not necessary.

There is also some disagreement about the usage of Reiki boosters among Reiki Masters. Some Masters advertise that free booster attunements are available to their students upon request whenever they wish. However, not all Reiki Masters offer booster attunements to their students. They feel that the initial classroom attunements are sufficient. According to their way of thinking, as long as practitioners are faithful to practicing Reiki, their ki channels will remain open and free of blockages. They believe that whenever Reiki is done routinely, there is no need for anyone to request a booster attunement to clear the body.

A Reiki Master might feel that the practitioner who requests a booster attunement is lazy, does not practice Reiki faithfully, wants his body to be cleared of blockages "the easy way," or is simply a compulsive "energy junkie" or "energy thrill-seeker." Indeed, experiencing an attunement can be a thrill. There is no argument among Reiki Masters that an attunement can induce a joyous experience.

Long-Distance Attunements

A new practice, which has emerged with the upsurge in the popularity of the Internet, is receiving Reiki attunements via "long-distance Reiki." There are currently videotapes available on the market through which you can supposedly receive your Reiki attunement electronically while watching and listening to a preprogrammed attunement.

Whether or not this type of long-distance attunement actually qualifies as a valid attunement is a frequently debated issue. Some people have reported that they have experienced attunements both ways, hands-on and long distance, and that both procedures were equally effective. Furthermore, many practitioners claim that it is reasonable to assume that if Reiki treatments can be conducted at long distance, passing long-distance attunements should be possible as well.

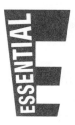

A Reiki attunement should not be viewed as a "magic bullet." The attunement merely opens or awakens the body so that the practitioner can serve as a conduit for Reiki energies to flow through. An attunement does not make a proficient practitioner or fix misaligned chakras. Routine Reiki self-treatments improve a practitioner's ability to become adept as a healer and helps to keep his or her chakras open and functioning.

A problem that many people have with some of the long-distance attunements advertised is that they are being conducted by individuals who haven't been trained to pass them in this manner. At one time there was even a hyperlink on an Internet Web page that read, "Click here to become a Reiki Master." After the Web page was opened, the following words appeared on the computer monitor screen: "Congratulations, you are now a Reiki Master." Whether done in jest, as a hoax, or as a statement of sarcasm by a Reiki skeptic, this Web page could be harmful, especially to people who may have taken it seriously. This absurd example gives one sufficient cause to question the effectiveness of a long-distance attunement compared to one passed hands-on.

How certain can you be that the person who attunes you over the Internet is a legitimate Reiki Master/Teacher? Is it more likely that you would be deceived by a teacher you meet on the Internet and only communicate with through e-mails or by a teacher you meet in person and converse with face-to-face? There are no right or wrong answers implied here, but these are questions worth thinking about.

Sending Absentia Reiki Energies

Most practitioners will agree that it is important to get permission before sending absentia Reiki energies. But, how that permission is obtained is up for discussion within the Reiki community. Some Reiki practitioners will agree to send a distance treatment to someone in response to a request made by a family member or a friend. If such is the case, the practitioner will send distance Reiki with an attached intention statement indicating that the energies he or she sends are available if the recipient's subconscious mind or soul is willing and open to receiving them.

But not all Reiki practitioners agree. Some practitioners will never send distant Reiki treatments without receiving a verbal or written request directly from the recipient. For them, a request made by a family member or a friend isn't enough. They feel that it is not an ethical way to send Reiki, because it is somehow deceitful. In their minds, it's like offering a prayer on behalf of another person without that person's consent. This makes sense to some people, but not to others. Millions of people worldwide do pray for others without first obtaining their consent for prayer. The bottom line is, it's your call. Reiki will honor either choice.

Sentiments over Symbols

Perhaps the most heated debates among Reiki practitioners are those in regard to the Reiki symbols. The symbols, when revealed to students, are supposed to be kept confidential. The drawings and the mantras are not to be used outside of passing attunements or giving treatments because of the power they possess. The caution given to students regarding the symbols might remind you of the warnings that children receive from their parents to avoid danger, like when they are instructed not to play with matches. In a similar manner, students are taught that misusing the Reiki symbols may lead to undesirable consequences.

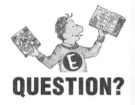

QUESTION?

Should the Power symbol be drawn counterclockwise?
The traditional Cho Ku Rei, Reiki's Power symbol, is drawn counterclockwise to increase power. However, there is dispute among some practitioners about the correctness of this procedure. A few practitioners feel that drawing the Cho Ku Rei symbol counterclockwise actually diminishes its power. Consequently, they have chosen to draw it clockwise.

What happens when a child is told not to play with a powerful toy unless under close supervision of his or her parent? The responses can be different, depending on the personality of the child. One child might agree never to play with the toy while alone. Another child might be too curious to keep away from the toy and will play with it when no one is around to supervise. Similarly, it became too difficult for certain practitioners to use their symbols in a few limited settings and to keep the Reiki symbols all to themselves.

One of the first reported occasions when the symbols were shared was at a retreat gathering that was attended by several of Takata's initiated Masters shortly after her death. Several of them began talking about the various symbols and drew them out on paper for each other to compare among their own drawings. They soon discovered that the symbols Takata had given to each of them were not exactly the same. The symbols as they had learned them were similar, but they had some variation to them.

Some of Takata's Masters went home and told their Reiki students what they had learned about Takata's symbols and how varied they were among the Masters. Students were told to continue to honor the sacredness of the symbols and not to share their personal symbols beyond the ranks of other Reiki II and Master Level practitioners. This meant that they no longer had to keep the symbols completely private, but that they could go ahead and share them with other practitioners.

The Cat's Out of the Bag

Before long, the symbols were leaked to the general public through books and over the Internet. The most noteworthy of these leaks was through the publication of Diane Stein's book *Essential Reiki: A Complete Guide to an Ancient Healing Art.* The boat is still rocking over the controversy triggered by that event!

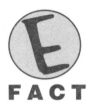

FACT

Stein was not surprised with how much controversy her book sparked. In fact, she had warned her readers that her revelations would be met with controversy. Even today, some Reiki practitioners are still angry with Stein for breaking the silence and sharing the Reiki symbols with the world.

Out of fear of Reiki's sacred symbols being exposed, some Masters began teaching that each practitioner's symbol carried its own "energy," based on the way it was placed in the student's crown and drawn on the student's dominant hand during the attunement rite. Each student was told that if she attempted to use another person's symbols, rather than the ones she had been shown, those symbols would have no power. Only the symbols that were passed to the student during the attunement would work. And it was further explained that if a person who had never been attuned to Reiki attempted to use the symbols, he would fail, because the symbols carried absolutely no power in and of themselves.

Real Power or Symbolic Representation?

Some Reiki practitioners continue to hold to the belief that Reiki's power is housed within the symbols. They feel that extreme care should be taken whenever using the symbols. Other practitioners feel that the symbols are only symbolic and that the power represented by the symbols is merely reflected by the practitioner's intent when using them. Whether or not you believe that healing powers are housed within the Reiki symbols is a matter of personal choice.

Making Up Your Mind

Reiki is a miraculous healing modality, but it is also a wonderful tool of self-discovery. Open discussions between Reiki practitioners over the several controversies that have arisen during the past years helps each of us recognize how we fit into the world with our differences and similarities. In the end, each of us is challenged to use our intelligence and gut feelings to best decide for ourselves what Reiki is and what it is not.

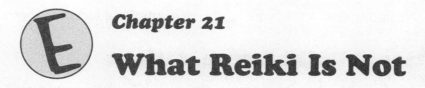

Chapter 21

What Reiki Is Not

Today there are more nontraditional Reiki Masters than traditional ones. Nontraditional Reiki Master/Teachers supplement their Reiki classes with teaching materials and techniques used in other healing methodologies. Some students come out of these nontraditional classes confused about what truly constitutes Reiki. Often the best way to define something is to describe in detail what that something is not.

What Reiki Is and Isn't	
Reiki Is . . .	Reiki Isn't . . .
A spiritual healing art	A religion
A way of life	A one-time cure
Energy work	Massage therapy
A complementary medicine	A substitute for medical care

Traditional Reiki Organizations

There is considerable confusion as to which Usui Reiki groups or Usui Reiki systems qualify as being traditional Reiki. Depending on whom you ask, the answers will vary considerably. Arguments can be made for and against many of these groups. Which of the following groups would you choose to regard as the most traditional?

- **Usui Reiki Ryoho Gakkai**—Usui Society in Japan
- **The Reiki Alliance**—Usui–Hayashi–Takata–Furumoto lineage
- **The Radiance Technique**—Barbara Weber Ray's seven degrees of Reiki, also known as Authentic Reiki and Real Reiki
- **Usui Shiki Ryoho**—All Usui Reiki practitioners who trained under Takata's lineage in the West, including the Reiki Alliance members as well as other practitioners

Usui Reiki Ryoho Gakkai

The Usui Reiki Ryoho Gakkai, founded by Dr. Mikao Usui, is still active today. This is primarily a secret society. It's likely that the Reiki they practice would be the closest to what Usui originally developed. However, the members do not use the term *traditional* to describe the Usui Reiki system they practice.

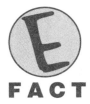

The Reiki certificate that Hawayo Takata was awarded by Chujiro Hayashi certified her as a Master of Dr. Usui's Reiki System of Healing. Her certificate was signed and notarized on February 21, 1938, in Honolulu, Hawaii. This certification qualified her as an Usui Reiki Master.

The Reiki Alliance

Members of the Reiki Alliance took it upon themselves to designate Phyllis Lei Furumoto as Takata's successor, awarding her the title of Reiki Grand Master. However, Takata never officially made Furumoto or anyone else her successor.

Some Reiki Alliance members don't consider those who have attained Reiki Master Level through non-Alliance Masters to be traditional Reiki Masters. Supposedly, these Alliance members are not happy that the nonmembers never paid the $10,000 fee for mastership as defined by Takata. There is still some controversy over which of these claims and allegations are true.

The Radiance Technique

In disagreement with Furumoto's claim, Barbara Weber Ray announced that she is the true successor to Takata. Ray asserts that Mrs. Takata gave her additional information, which no one else was made privy to. In particular, Takata passed on to her a teaching about the seven degrees of Reiki.

Ray was able to trademark her teachings as Authentic Reiki, also known as Real Reiki. Upon reviewing her Web site, the word *traditional* does not appear, but Ray does claim that she is the only person who was given the details of the entire Usui system. Considering Ray's viewpoint, one could assume that Ray and her Reiki initiates feel that they are following a traditional path.

Traditional or Not

Some traditional Reiki Masters have become disgruntled when other Reiki Masters, who supposedly do not qualify as traditional teachers, promote themselves as traditional Reiki Masters. They feel that any Reiki Master/Teacher who has strayed from Takata's teachings in any way at all should refer to himself or herself as a nontraditional or independent teacher.

However, recent research has revealed that Hayashi modified Usui's original teachings and that Takata also taught a modified form of Reiki that strayed from what Hayashi taught, perhaps to suit her own purposes. Considering these modifications in Reiki, discussions about who should or should not call themselves traditional teachers seem pointless.

Today, a widely accepted definition of a nontraditional Reiki Master/Teacher is someone who teaches the same basic principles that Takata taught her students, but who will also include instructions for additional healing methodologies in his or her Reiki class. A principled Reiki instructor will inform students that any additional techniques being taught in the classroom are not Reiki. Unfortunately, some Reiki teachers don't distinguish between these additional techniques and those of Reiki as clearly as they should. In other cases, students who do not pay close enough attention to instructions during a class might come out of the class assuming that these other ideas or techniques are a part of Reiki.

For these reasons, it has become difficult today to clearly express what is distinctly Reiki and what clearly is not Reiki. Just for the record, let's review the basics of traditional Reiki classes:

- Reiki history
- Reiki Principles
- Reiki attunements
- Reiki treatments
- Reiki hand placements
- Reiki symbols

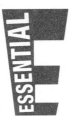

Many Reiki practitioners have acquired training in a variety of healing methods. For these practitioners, Reiki is only one of several tools tucked away in their medicine bags.

What Nontraditional Classes Have to Offer

Chapter 15 provides sample syllabuses of traditional Usui Reiki classes for the various levels of training. But perhaps you are more inclined to seek out a nontraditional Reiki Master in order to gather additional healing tools along with the attunements and Reiki training.

Because all Reiki classes are not equal, take your time researching nontraditional classes that are available. Also, if you are interested in specific healing methodologies like crystal therapy or chakra balancing, you may very well be able to find a Reiki Master who is adept in those areas as well.

On the Plus Side

Nontraditional teachers tend to have lower class fees. There are a few nontraditional teachers who even offer their services for free. If you take your time to carefully research and interview prospective nontraditional teachers, it is possible that you will find someone who has been attuned to Reiki, is very knowledgeable, and whose actions are well-principled.

On the Minus Side

If you don't bother to check up on a nontraditional teacher, you could be throwing your money away when he or she proves to be less than knowledgeable, or worse, fraudulent. Unfortunately, there are some charlatans out there who have never been attuned to Reiki and who offer bogus attunements to others. It's important to be on your guard! Some of these stinkers will even offer bogus attunements for free, simply for the thrill of deception.

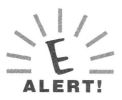

ALERT!

If you suspect that you have possibly received a fake attunement, don't blame yourself for being swindled. You are not the first to become a victim of a Reiki charlatan, and you will likely not be the last. Try to locate a reputable Reiki teacher in your area and begin your training over. All paths eventually lead to wisdom, including those we walk with misguided footsteps.

Distinguishing Reiki from Other Modalities

There are a wide variety of additional concepts taught in nontraditional Reiki classes. These methodologies and techniques are often combined with Reiki during a treatment. As a result, the recipient will walk away from this species of Reiki treatment thinking that Reiki consists of massage, crystal therapy, aromatherapy—the whole kit and caboodle. But nothing could be further from the truth.

If a recipient has come to you expecting a Reiki treatment, it is your obligation to conduct a Reiki treatment without the integration of other healing methods—unless those other methods have been mutually agreed upon. For example, if you are in the habit of combining the use of aromatherapy or flower essence therapy when giving Reiki treatments, your recipients may assume that essential oils or essences are a part of Reiki. Act responsibly and clarify what Reiki is, and what it is not, so that there will be no lingering confusion or doubt.

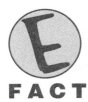

FACT

Reiki does not involve muscle manipulation, crystal therapy, psychic surgery, or chakra work. Although Reiki can be effectively combined with these and other healing methods, none of these things are Reiki.

Reiki and Other Healing Practices

It's important to make a distinction between Reiki and other methods of treatment, but there's no reason to separate Reiki from other healing practices. Moreover, if you are clearly relying on another healing treatment, it is not necessary to tell the recipient that Reiki is also involved. If you're giving a massage, you don't need to warn your client that you may use Reiki energies as well. For one thing, you may not actually plan to include Reiki in these types of sessions. However, Reiki has a mind of its own. It flows when and where it is needed.

Nurses and massage therapists who have been attuned to Reiki may never disclose when Reiki starts flowing from their palms as they handle their patients. Reiki will naturally "kick in" when it is needed and will continue to flow for as long as the recipient is subconsciously open to receiving it. Healers become accustomed to Reiki flowing freely from their hands as they perform their duties. They need not feel obligated to share this information. Hospice workers and nursing assistants who are Reiki practitioners will also notice Reiki flowing through them to the people they are assisting.

Staying on the Reiki Path

Reiki history is steeped in tradition. Some Reiki practitioners are questioning parts of the tradition that have been proved less than accurate. As a result, new ways of practicing Reiki are constantly evolving. Today, Reiki continues to thrive in the healing community because its healing aspects stand by themselves. Choosing to take a nontraditional path in the study of Reiki does have its merits. However, we need to be cautious, since it is likely that there will always be individuals who will misrepresent Reiki for their own self-interests.

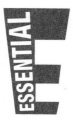

Types of modalities that Reiki can easily be integrated with include massage therapy, reflexology, acupuncture, chiropractic care, chakra alignment, polarity therapy, and regression therapy.

Reiki is *not* everything. Reiki is only one healing system, and, although it would likely take more than a lifetime for a person to say he or she fully understands the complexities within this simple healing art, there are many other hands-on healing systems worth exploring. It is good to be open to all possibilities!

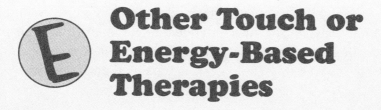

Chapter 22

Other Touch or Energy-Based Therapies

Aside from Reiki, there are many other therapies, both ancient and modern, that are based on "touch" and/or "life force." Each has its own unique history, purpose, and methodology. Techniques used in Healing Touch and Quantum-Touch are very closely related to Reiki. Hands-on healing modalities that are based on the use of ki energies, such as the Alexander Technique and shiatsu massage, involve manipulation of the body's bone structure, muscles, and skin.

Alexander Technique

The Alexander Technique is a body alignment therapy used to help recipients manage pain, relax muscular tension, learn corrective breathing techniques, and develop better postures.

This technique is based on the premise that tightened muscles support misaligned bone structure, expend unnecessary energy, and create discomfort and fatigue. The Alexander Technique teacher uses his or her hands to gently release muscular strains and encourage correction of the bone structure so that the whole body is balanced and in good alignment.

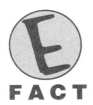

FACT

Australian singer and actor Frederick Matthias Alexander (1869–1955) developed the Alexander Technique as a result of pursuing pain relief for his vocal and throat problems.

The recipient becomes an active participant in the treatment through body awareness, acquiring better posture and body movement habits— which, in turn, allow the skeletal structure to align naturally with the relaxed muscles.

Aura Clearing and Chakra Balancing

Many different techniques have been introduced in recent years that can be employed to clean "dirty" auras and correct "imbalanced" chakras. Three highly respected healers who have participated in extensive studies involving the human energy field are Rosalyn L. Bruyere, Caroline Myss, Ph.D., and Barbara Ann Brennan. Each of these women has the intuitive ability to see a person's energy field, including their aura and chakra system. Together, Bruyere, Myss, and Brennan authored several books on the subject of auras and chakras. Recently, many healers have been showing interest in the study of the chakras and the human energy field.

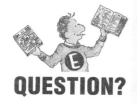
QUESTION?

What are the chakras?
Also known as energy vortexes or wheels of light, chakras are funnel-shaped centers within our bodies that serve as intake and outflow mechanisms to control the flow of ki energies that sustain us. Open and functioning chakras spin clockwise, allowing energy to vitalize our auras and nourish our physical bodies. Healers are familiar with seven major and twenty-one minor chakras.

First Chakra

The first chakra, also known as the root chakra, is associated with the color red. This chakra is the grounding force that allows us to connect to the earth energies and empowers our life force. It is through this chakra that the child feels a connection with his or her birth mother and also the nuclear family. This area is also the place from which our survival instincts spring forth. When this chakra is misaligned, we experience confusion, distraction, and disconnection.

Second Chakra

The second chakra, also known as the sacral chakra, is associated with the colors orange and red-orange. This chakra often offers us the opportunity to acknowledge our issues regarding control, especially regarding our relationships with others. The process of creating changes in our lives through making personal choices is a function of second chakra energy. A well-functioning second chakra helps a person maintain a healthy yin-yang existence.

Third Chakra

The third chakra, also known as the solar plexus chakra, is associated with the color yellow. This is where our egos and intuitions reside. The healthfulness or lack of healthfulness of this chakra shapes our personal self-esteem. If you experience difficulty maintaining your personal power, it's a telltale sign that your third chakra is compromised. This intuitive chakra is also the source from which we get those "gut feelings" that signal us to take action or to avoid something. Our intuitive skills are sharpened when this chakra is functioning optimally.

Fourth Chakra

The fourth chakra, also known as the heart chakra, is associated with the colors green or pink. This chakra is considered to be the love center of our human energy system. Physical illnesses that are brought about by wounds of the heart require that an emotional healing occur along with the physical healing. Our deepest emotions, such as love, heartbreak, grief, pain, and fear, are felt strongly in this chakra. For this reason, energy-based therapies that focus on balancing the heart chakra are often the purest healing. Learning self-love is a powerful initiative to undertake in order to secure a healthy fourth chakra.

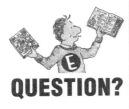

QUESTION?

What are the yin and yang?
Yin reflects the passive, nonmoving, feminine energies. Yang reflects the active, moving, masculine energies. Yin-yang is the Chinese philosophy that opposites are complementary. The yin-yang aspects of our mind and body must be in balance to assure optimum health and well-being.

Fifth Chakra

The fifth chakra, also known as the throat chakra, is associated with the color sky-blue. This chakra is our will center. It is through our speech that we express ourselves to others. The healthfulness of the fifth chakra is signified by how honestly a person expresses himself or herself. A challenge to the throat chakra is for us to express ourselves in the most truthful manner. When we choose to speak falsehoods and half-truths, we are energetically polluting the throat chakra and violating both our bodies and spirits. Repressing our anger or displeasure by ignoring these emotions through evasive sweet talk, or keeping silent, will manifest into throat imbalances such as strep throat, laryngitis, speech impediments, etc.

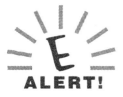

ALERT!

Divorce or separation, grief due to death, emotional abuse, abandonment, and adultery are all examples of hurtful situations that can affect our emotional well-being. All of these can wound the heart chakra.

We have all experienced that lump in our throat at times when we are unable to find the right words to speak. But when the words do begin to form, it is important that we project them clearly and truthfully with our voices. When we do not speak out, we are not only stifling our speech, but we are also stifling our heartfelt emotions. All choices we make in our lives have consequences on an energetic level, even our silences. Doing nothing and saying nothing are life choices that can affect our health.

Sixth Chakra

The sixth chakra, also known as the brow chakra, is associated with the color indigo. It is also often referred to as either the third eye or the mind center. Our mental calculations and thinking processes are functions of this chakra. We are able to evaluate our past experiences and put them into perspective through the wisdom of this chakra's actions.

Our ability to separate reality from fantasy or delusion is connected to the healthfulness of this chakra. Achieving the art of detachment outside the frame of petty-mindedness is accomplished through developing impersonal intuitive reasoning. It is through a receptive brow chakra that aura colors and other visual images are intuitively received.

Seventh Chakra

The seventh chakra, also known as the crown chakra, is associated with the color violet or white. The crown chakra is used as a mechanism for inner communication with our spiritual nature. The opening in the crown chakra serves as an entryway wherein the Universal Life Force can enter our bodies and be dispersed downward into the lower six chakras.

This chakra is often depicted as a lotus flower with its petals open to represent spiritual awakening. The crown chakra could also be considered the bottomless well from which intuitive knowledge is drawn.

Bowen Therapy

The Bowen technique was originally developed and practiced by an Australian named Thomas Ambrose Bowen (1903–1982). Bowen Therapy is a gentle, relaxing bodywork that is administered by manipulating thumb and fingers in a rolling motion over muscles to release energy blocks. Waiting periods are incorporated between sequenced series of movements, which are conducted across specific muscle and connective tissues to alleviate different physical dis-eases. The precise, delicate movements are applied to the recipient's muscles, either directly over the skin or through light clothing. It is reported that Bowen Therapy may help to relieve the following conditions:

- Autoimmune diseases
- Digestive disorders
- Gynecological problems
- Musculoskeletal pain
- Respiratory problems

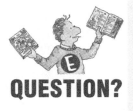

QUESTION?

Is Bowen Therapy difficult to learn?
Gerri Shapiro, MS Ed., health educator and Bowen practitioner, developed a videotape, titled *Miracle Pain Relief—The Gentle Power of Bowen*, which demonstrates the Bowen technique in easy-to-follow steps. She uses terminology that is understandable for beginners.

Healing Touch

Healing Touch was developed by Janet Mentgen, RN, BSN. In 1990, this program of study was accepted as a certificate program of the American

Holistic Nurses Association (AHNA). The Canadian Holistic Nurses Association has endorsed it as well. In 1996, Healing Touch International, Inc., became the certifying organization for this hands-on energy-based therapy.

Healing Touch consists of six levels of training, Level I, IIA, IIB, III, IV, and V. Each level requires a commitment of several hours of instruction to gain knowledge and hands-on practice to develop Healing Touch skill. Practitioner certification can be attained after Level III. Level IV training is for the practitioner's involvement in case studies, mentoring others, and establishing client/therapist relationship, ethics, and development of a private practice. Level V is the instructor level, intended for the certified Healing Touch practitioner to learn how to teach Healing Touch.

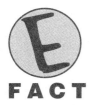

FACT

Healing Touch is practiced outside of the United States as well. In fact, Healing Touch International, Inc., has certified Healing Touch practitioners from Canada, Australia, New Zealand, and The Netherlands.

Huna Healing

Huna Healing is more than a healing therapy. In addition to its healing properties, Huna is also a principled way of life. Huna Healing is an ancient energy-work system that originated in the Hawaiian Islands. Its name, attributed to Max Freedom Long, is Hawaiian for "secret."

In its purest form, Huna Healing is ancient knowledge enabling a person to connect to his or her highest wisdom within. Understanding and utilizing the fundamentals, or Seven Principles, of Huna can help people bring about healing and harmony through the power of the mind. As an integrated healing art and earth culture, Huna is spiritual in nature. Experiencing its concepts gives us the opportunity to integrate mind, body, and spirit. One might acknowledge Huna teachings as one of nature's tools helpful in developing inner knowledge and enhancing innate psychic abilities.

Seven Principles of Huna	
Ike	The world is what you think it is.
Kala	There are no limits. Everything is possible.
Makia	Energy flows where attention goes.
Manawa	Now is the moment of power.
Aloha	To love is to be happy with.
Mana	All power comes from within.
Pono	Effectiveness is the measure of truth.

Johrei Healing

Johrei healing is a Japanese focusing and scanning technique used to dispel negativity and to increase vitality. No actual touching is involved in this healing process.

The Johrei practitioner and recipient sit in chairs facing one another. The practitioner holds the palm of her hand toward the recipient while focusing and directing ki energies toward him. Energies are directed at the recipient's forehead, upper chest, and abdomen for approximately ten minutes. Then the recipient is asked to face the opposite direction, with his back to the Johrei practitioner. The practitioner focuses and directs ki energies toward the recipient's crown and the back of his head, then toward both shoulders and down the spine. Finally, the recipient returns to his original sitting position so that they are once again facing each other. The two individuals, practitioner and recipient, join together and give a silent prayer of gratitude.

The following positive effects are attributed to Johrei healing:

- It increases spiritual quality of life.
- It clears mental confusion.
- It detoxifies the physical body.
- It accelerates the process of healing.

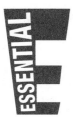

The Johrei Fellowship Web site (✑www.johreifoundation.org) shares the beliefs of the fellowship. According to it, "Any individual, when properly prepared, can focus this universal energy. The intensity may differ according to the level of the individual's awareness, but it is possible for any individual to focus it effectively."

Johrei healing is only one aspect of the Johrei Fellowship, which is a spiritually principled organization. Johrei was introduced to America in 1953, and Johrei Fellowship centers exist throughout the United States. The fellowship has incorporated the following Seven Spiritual Principles into its work:

1. Order
2. Gratitude
3. Purification
4. Spiritual affinity
5. Cause and effect
6. The spiritual precedes the physical
7. Oneness of the spiritual and the physical

Polarity Therapy

Randolph Stone, DO, DC, ND (1890–1981), developed Polarity Therapy. In 1984, a national organization, the American Polarity Therapy Association, was established to practice and teach this healing system.

Polarity Therapy involves energy-based bodywork, nutrition, exercise, and self-awareness. The Polarity Therapy practitioner assesses the recipient's energetic attributes using touch, observation, and interview methods. Application of touching can range from light touch to medium or firm pressure. The techniques used in this therapy are complementary to many other holistic health systems.

Pranic Healing

Pranic Healing is a nontouch energy-based technique that accelerates the healing process through the use of "life-force" being directed to the part of the physical body that needs healing. In order to locate blockages of ki, the Pranic practitioner scans the recipient's aura or "energy field." Ki energies are then projected through the Pranic practitioner's palm chakras to cleanse, energize, and revitalize the problematic area.

Grand Master Choa Kok Sui founded Pranic Healing as a result of spending over eighteen years researching and studying esoteric sciences. He has written several books about his findings, including *Miracles through Pranic Healing* and *Advanced Pranic Healing*.

Stephen Co is a senior disciple of Grand Master Choa Kok Sui and the world's foremost authority Pranic Healing. In his Pranic Healing workshops, Co teaches a simple exercise that activates the palm chakras.

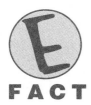

FACT

VortexHealing is a spiritually oriented healing system that is based on the premise that all of our ailments are the result of us experiencing separation from the divine consciousness. In 1995, Ric Weinman, founder of VortexHealing, began teaching this healing art in order to assist the process of spiritual awakening.

Shiatsu Massage

Shiatsu, also known as acupressure, is a finger pressure massage technique that is sometimes confused with acupuncture. Although both shiatsu massage therapy and acupuncture are founded on the Chinese meridian system, there are no needle pokes involved with shiatsu. Massage techniques like tapping, squeezing, rubbing, and applied pressure are applied along the meridians to reintroduce the optimal flow of ki.

Energy Pathways

Meridians are the pathways of ki and blood flow through the body. When a person's overall health is good, ki will flow continuously from one meridian to another. Any break in the flow is an indication of imbalance. Whenever a person's vitality or energy is recognizably diminished, this signifies that the body's organs or tissues are functioning poorly and, therefore, the ki flow is insufficient.

The Meridian Healing System

The meridian healing system is based on the concept that an insufficient supply of ki compromises a person's immune system, making him or her vulnerable to dis-ease. Restoring the ki is the ultimate goal in restoring overall health and well-being to the individual. Acupuncturists, Chinese herbalists, and shiatsu massage therapists assist clients in repairing dysfunctional areas within the meridian system in order to restore a natural balance.

Twelve Major Meridians

There are twelve major meridians, which correspond to specific human organs: kidneys, liver, spleen, heart, lungs, pericardium, bladder, gall bladder, stomach, small and large intestines, and the triple burner (body temperature regulator). Yin meridians flow upward. Yang meridians flow downward. Pathways corresponding to the yang organ are often used to treat disorders of its related yin organ.

Corresponding Yin and Yang Organs	
Yin Organs	**Yang Organs**
Lungs	Large intestine
Pericardium	Triple burner
Heart	Small intestine
Spleen	Stomach
Liver	Gallbladder
Kidney	Bladder

Therapeutic Touch

Therapeutic Touch is considered a modern version of an array of ancient energy-based healing methods. Dolores Krieger, Ph.D., RN, and Dora Van Gelder Kunz developed this healing system. Therapeutic Touch was originally taught to a group of graduate nurses in 1972 and today is still primarily practiced among health care professionals. However, the training is not exclusive to nurses and doctors—it is also available to anyone else who wishes to learn it.

A basic Therapeutic Touch workshop consists of approximately twelve classroom hours. To qualify as a Therapeutic Touch practitioner, a student must take the intermediate-level workshop and be mentored for twelve months under the care of a qualified Therapeutic Touch practitioner/teacher.

The Therapeutic Touch practitioner applies gentle sweeping movements with his or her hands a few inches over the body to clear away imbalances and revitalize the recipient's personal energy. Its primary purposes are to manage pain and promote healing.

The Trager Approach

The Trager Approach is a tension-reducing treatment involving gentle rocking and vibrating movements. The intention of a Trager treatment is to release built-up patterns of tension in the joints and muscles of the body, creating a sense of deep relaxation within the recipient. The recipient remains passive throughout the process and is encouraged to relax and "let go" physically, mentally, and emotionally. Following treatment, simple exercises called "Mentastics" are given to the recipient for home use. These exercises are meant to reinforce the subconscious messages initiated during treatment.

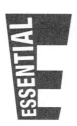

The Trager Approach has been reported to ease or manage a wide range of conditions, including stress, back and neck pain, limited movement, muscle spasms, depression, headaches, multiple sclerosis, postpolio syndrome, cerebral palsy, sports-related injuries, Parkinson's disease, carpal tunnel syndrome, and fibromyalgia.

Milton Trager, M.D. (1908–1997), who developed the Trager Approach, became interested in the structure and function of the body as a result of a childhood congenital spinal deformity he overcame. In 1980, Trager established the Trager Institute with the help of Betty Fuller.

Quantum-Touch

Quantum-Touch is a vibrational touch therapy that incorporates touch, breath work, and body awareness meditations. Its concepts are closely related to polarity therapy. It is primarily a light-touch energy therapy, but it is secondarily promoted as a therapy that helps bones to spontaneously adjust to their proper alignment. Richard Gordon developed Quantum-Touch therapy and published a book on this therapy, *Quantum-Touch: The Power to Heal.*

The Quantum-Touch healing process involves the practitioner "running energy" into the recipient's body. Often, practitioners employ a technique that is known as "sandwiching" or "the hand sandwich." Sandwiching means that the practitioner will use his or her hands to sandwich the part of the recipient's body that is to be treated. One hand will be placed on one side of the body part and the other hand will be placed on the other side. Another technique that is used for "running energy" into very small areas is to create a tripod using the thumb, forefinger, and middle finger. This is meant to help get the practitioner's hands closer to the source of pain. Advanced techniques used in this system include harmonic toning, spinning the chakras, structural alignment, and distant healing. Ⓔ

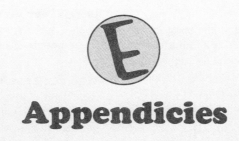

Appendicies

Appendix A

Frequently Asked
Questions

Appendix B

Glossary of Terms

Appendix C

Additional Resources

Appendix A

Frequently Asked Questions

What is Reiki?

Reiki is a natural healing system designed to assist in healing and help achieve balance. Reiki is administered by a practitioner, who serves as a conduit through whom the Universal Life Energy can be transmitted to the recipient, by either hands-on or distance healing techniques. Practitioners may also practice Reiki self-treatments.

How does Reiki energy flow?

Reiki flows through our palms at different rates of speed, depending on various factors such as the extent of the recipient's illness, degree of blockage, his or her readiness to accept change, and so on.

How can I best understand Reiki?

The best way to understand and appreciate Reiki is to experience it by having a full-body Reiki treatment. Reiki is for everyone and it is available to anyone who wants it.

Is Reiki a form of faith healing?

No, Reiki is not a religion, nor is it based on the acceptance of any religious doctrine. Having a belief system is not a requirement for Reiki to work. Reiki does not infringe on anyone's right to believe what he or she wishes. However, Reiki's principles are spiritual in nature and do encourage spiritual empowerment and growth.

Can Reiki be learned from a book?

Becoming a Reiki practitioner is not something you can do on your own through reading a how-to book or watching an instructional video. Receiving Reiki attunements and training can be achieved in a one-day or two-day workshop. Access to Reiki is easy. All you have to do is seek out a Reiki Master in your area who is willing to work with you.

Is Reiki for everyone?

Reiki is for everyone, but not everyone is for Reiki. Some people are simply not as open to Reiki as others.

Who can benefit from a Reiki treatment?

Reiki's gift of increased energy and vitality can be extended to anyone. It doesn't matter what a person's gender, race, intelligence, or financial status is. Reiki is not a healing energy reserved only for the elite, wealthy, educated, or spiritually evolved.

What does Reiki feel like?

Common Reiki sensations are heat or coolness, "pins and needles" tingling, vibrational buzzing, electrical sparks, numbness, throbbing, itchiness, and drowsiness.

What is a Reiki attunement?

A Reiki attunement is a ritual performed by a Reiki Master. The ritual involves energetic placement of Reiki symbols, through a specific set of sequenced actions, into the student's crown and palms.

What types of changes can I expect following my Reiki attunement?

Changes will vary from person to person, so it's impossible to predict how any one individual will react to being attuned. Changes begin to take place as soon as Reiki is introduced into the body and begins its balancing process. Reiki works to bring about only positive changes, but these changes may offer challenges while the transformation is occurring.

Will I know when Reiki is working?

Some people know when Reiki is working because they notice shifts of energies occurring. However, some people don't feel anything when giving or receiving Reiki. Just because you don't feel anything, don't assume nothing is happening. Trust that Reiki is working.

What if my hands don't feel hot?

Experiencing hot hands is a common experience reported by Reiki practitioners. However, each person's experience with Reiki is unique. You may not experience hot hands, so don't look for it as verification that Reiki is flowing through them.

I feel balls of energy collecting in my hands. What is that all about?

When excess Reiki energies build up in your palms, it may be an indication that a Reiki self-treatment is needed. Take advantage of this excess of energy in your hands and place your hands on your body. Allowing the Reiki to flow into your body should help reduce or release the ball of energy from your palms.

Will Reiki ever run out?

When you are giving a Reiki treatment to someone, you are giving of your time and your intent to assist, but you are not giving away any of your own energy. Reiki is in infinite supply. It never runs out.

Does nutrition play a role in Reiki?

Definitely! Having optimal health is essential for practicing Reiki, and eating nutritional meals regularly is essential for optimal health. Eating five or six small-portion meals each day is recommended over eating just two or three large meals.

What is the purpose of the Reiki hand placements?

Emphasis is placed on devoting five minutes on each hand placement so that no part of the body is neglected and to ensure that each body part is given equal consideration. After practicing these twelve hand placements in the traditional sequences for a period of time, you will likely deviate from them to some degree and begin to acquire your own methodology in placing your hands on your body while listening to your inner dialogue.

How often should I conduct self-treatments?

Newly attuned Reiki Level I practitioners will benefit from doing full-body sessions daily for the first four to six weeks. After those first weeks, following a regimen of one or two full-body self-treatments each week is prudent.

Are there any limitations to Reiki?

The only limitations that can block Reiki are those we create, consciously or subconsciously, through a lack of trust or belief in the potential of Reiki treatments to improve our balance or conditions of health.

Do I need to direct the flow of Reiki?

Reiki will automatically go to wherever it needs to go with no mental involvement of either the practitioner or the recipient. However, when mental intention is used, a linear pathway is opened. This cleared route allows Reiki to flow more effectively to that part of the body where attention is most desired.

Now that I'm a Reiki practitioner, am I obligated to treat others?

You are under no obligation to treat others every time it is requested of you. You have the right to refuse treatment to anyone, without justifying your feelings. Anytime you feel strongly that you do not want to give a Reiki treatment to someone, accept those feelings without hesitation and politely refuse.

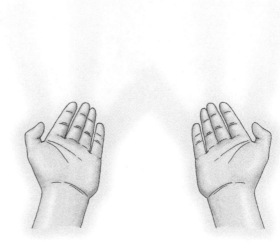

What purpose do Reiki symbols serve?

Independently, each Reiki symbol has its own unique purposes. The combined function of these symbols is to provide Reiki practitioners with focal points for their healing intentions.

Why is Reiki called "smart energy"?

Reiki is an intelligent energy because it knows which areas of the body most need healing and will automatically flow to specific areas where suffering or imbalance are prevalent.

What is a Reiki share?

A Reiki share is a time when Reiki practitioners gather together to socialize and to participate in group healing treatments. The main purpose of the share is to give and receive Reiki in a casual atmosphere of friendship, honor, and devotion.

Why did I start crying during my Reiki treatment?

Occasionally a person will experience an intense emotional release during or after a Reiki treatment. These types of emotional release may be expressed through crying, screaming, coughing, vomiting, or other reactions. Emotional releases help carry the person through the hurts and discomforts associated with the feelings that arise during a Reiki session.

Why is it important to sweep the recipient's auric field after a Reiki treatment?

Sweeping or combing through the recipient's auric field clears it of any energetic debris that has lifted from the physical body during the treatment. It is also recommended that you clear your healing space between Reiki treatments so that you don't have any negative or stagnant energies lingering in any part of the room.

Is it safe to treat children with Reiki?

Reiki's gentle and noninvasive nature is perfect for treating the ills and upsets of young children. Children are extremely receptive to Reiki's positive effects and will normally welcome it without any apprehension.

How important is it to attain the Master Level of training?

Being certified in the highest level does not necessarily reflect superior knowledge. It is through the continued practice of Reiki that one becomes proficient. The Level I practitioner who uses Reiki daily will be more aware of how Reiki works than a Level III or Master Level Reiki practitioner who seldom conducts treatments.

Glossary of Terms

absentia treatment
A specially formulated Reiki treatment applied whenever treating an individual or group of individuals who are not physically present. A variety of items can be used as focal points while sending an absentia treatment: healing lists, photographs, teddy bear surrogates, and so forth. Absentia treatment is also known as distant healing or long-distance healing.

Advanced Reiki Training (ART)
This is the third level of training, also called Level IIIa, of the Usui/Tibetan Reiki System. ART consists of a variety of add-on techniques such as the use of crystal grids, spirit guides, healing attunements, psychic surgeries, meditations, and Tibetan symbols.

Akashic Records
People who believe in reincarnation believe that all lifetimes—past, present, and future—are recorded and are constantly being updated. These recordings are stored in the Akashic Records, which supposedly exists in an etheric dimension beyond the earth's atmosphere. It is said that everything that has ever happened since the beginning of time (every event, every thought, every action, every feeling) is recorded there. The term *akasha* is derived from the Sanskrit for "ether." Akashic Records are also known as Akasha Chronicles or Akashic Library.

attunement
Attunement is the empowerment ritual used to awaken the Reiki energies that lie dormant in everyone's body at birth. Reiki symbols are placed into the attunee's crown and palms. It is through the attunement process that Reiki is passed from teacher to student. Attunement may also be referred to as empowerment or initiation.

booster attunements
Booster attunements are Reiki attunements that are given to a Reiki practitioner as a "turbo charge" to help get the Reiki flowing whenever it is dormant or blocked. The Reiki Master can use the Hui Yin attunement as a booster attunement for any level practitioner.

Byosen Reikan Ho
Byosen Reikan Ho is a scanning technique that is used to detect dis-eases and imbalances, including those that have not yet manifested in the body. It is also used to treat residual toxins from past illnesses and as a preventative measure against the reoccurrence of past illnesses.

chakras
Also known as energy vortexes or wheels of light, chakras are funnel-shaped centers within our bodies that serve as intake and outflow mechanisms to control the flow of ki energies that sustain us. Open and functioning chakras spin clockwise, allowing energy to vitalize our auras and nourish our physical bodies. There are seven major chakras and twenty-one minor chakras.

Cho Ku Rei
This is the first symbol used in Reiki. It is generally called the Power symbol. In hands-on treatments, the Cho Ku Rei is often applied by tracing it in the air counterclockwise in order to increase power. Some practitioners also draw or visualize it in a clockwise motion, to decrease the flow of energy. The Cho Ku Rei symbol can be applied to help get the Reiki "juices" flowing when the energy flow has slowed down or become blocked. When it is used for absentia healings, it is drawn or visualized to act as the "Light Switch" that turns the Reiki on.

Dai Ko Myo

This is the Reiki symbol that represents the Usui Master symbol; it is also known as a Soul Healer. It is revealed to the Reiki student at the third-degree level.

Dumo

The Dumo is a Tibetan symbol used in attunement in the Usui Tibetan Reiki System. Its purpose is to ignite the Kundalini flame that is located in the root chakra. The Dumo is also known as the Tibetan Master symbol or the Tibetan Dai Ko Myo.

Gakkai

The Usui Reiki Ryoho Gakkai was the original Reiki organization that Dr. Mikao Usui founded in Japan. It is still active today. In Japanese, *gakkai* means "society."

Gassho

The Gassho is a prayerlike acknowledgment of the god or goddess spirit within each of us. The Gassho is also known as the Namaste.

Hatsurei ho

This is a meditation and breathing technique that was used by Dr. Mikao Usui and is still used in Reiki Ryoho as practiced by the Japanese Gakkai. Its purpose is to empower practitioners by increasing and enhancing their Reiki channel and their connection to the Universal Life Force.

Hon Sha Ze Sho Nen

The Hon Sha Ze Sho Nen is the third symbol used in Reiki. Primary functions of this symbol are sending absentia treatments, inner-child work, healing addictions, and reviewing Akashic Records. This symbol is also known as the Pagoda symbol and the Connection symbol.

Hui Yin Position

The Reiki Master holds this position when passing attunements. The vaginal muscles and anus are contracted, blocking air from entering the vagina and rectum. While holding the Hui Yin, the tongue is pressed against the roof of the mouth, with the tip of the tongue slightly touching the gap between the back of the two front teeth. A deep breath is taken and held for two to four minutes.

kanji

Modified Chinese characters used in the Japanese writing system; Reiki symbols are derived from kanji. Kanji characters are pictograms that represent entire ideas or words, rather than merely alphabet letters or syllables of words.

ki

The life force or living energy that connects us to all there is and sustains our life breath. While the Chinese refer to the life force as chi, or *qi,* in Japan this living energy that connects us to all there is and that sustains our life breath is called *ki.* The Hindus know it as *prana,* the Greeks as *pneuma,* the Polynesians as *mana,* and the Egyptians as *ka.*

Kundalini

Literally "coiled," like a bedspring, the Kundalini is considered to be the creative energy housed at the base of the spine. As the Kundalini is awakened and moves upward through the chakra system, a person's consciousness changes. Kundalini is also referred to as the Fire Serpent.

Okuden

In the traditional Japanese system of Reiki, Okuden is the equivalent to Usui Reiki Level II in the Western teachings.

practitioner

All levels of Reiki attunees are referred to as Reiki practitioners, meaning that they practice Reiki. You can also refer to Reiki practitioners as healers or Reiki facilitators.

Radiance Technique

This is one Reiki system that was born out of Hawayo Takata's teachings. Barbara Weber Ray, one of Takata's twenty-two initiates, developed this technique using secret information that she claims was entrusted to her by Takata before her death in 1980. Radiance Technique is also trademarked as Real Reiki and Authentic Reiki.

Raku

This Reiki symbol is used to finalize the attunement process. Its purpose is to lock the newly added energies within the Reiki initiate. The Raku is also known as the Lightning Bolt and the Completion symbol.

Reiho

An abbreviated name for Reiki Ryoho, or Reiki-ho, the practices and system used in the Usui Reiki Ryoho Gakkai.

Reiji

This is the intuitive ability to locate imbalances in the body without touching it. The person's hands are intuitively led to areas and specific spots on which to lay their hands in order to facilitate a healing. This is the technique that was taught in Japan to Reiki students before the hand placements were developed.

Reiju

Reiju is the original empowerment or initiation process used by Dr. Mikao Usui to pass Reiki energy on to his students. Reiju eventually developed into the Reiki attunement process that is recognized in the West.

The Reiki Alliance

The Reiki Alliance is an international community of Reiki Masters of Usui Shiki Ryoho that was formed in 1983. The Reiki Alliance acknowledges the lineage of Mikao Usui, Chujiro Hayashi, Hawayo Takata, and Phyllis Lei Furumoto.

Reiki Principles

A series of five principles, creeds, or precepts written by the Meiji Emperor that were adopted by Usui in Reiki Ryoho. There are many different variations of these five basic principles used by Reiki practitioners today.

Sei Hei Ki

Sei Hei Ki is the second Reiki symbol. Its purposes include emotional healings, purification, clearing, and protection. It is also known as the Dragon and the Harmony symbol.

sensei

A Japanese word for "teacher."

Shinpiden

In the traditional Japanese system of Reiki, Shinpiden is the equivalent to Usui Reiki Master/Teacher Level in the Western teachings.

Shoden

In the traditional Japanese system of Reiki, Shoden is the equivalent to Usui Reiki Level I in the Western teachings.

Usui Shiki Ryoho

The Japanese system of natural healing that originated from the Reiki System of Healing, as developed by Dr. Mikao Usui. It was adopted and further adapted by Chujiro Hayashi and Hawayo Takata. Usui Shiki Ryoho has since evolved into many different Reiki healing systems that draw from the same energy source.

Appendix C

Additional Resources

Further Readings

Books

All Love: A Guidebook for Healing With Sekhem-Seichim-Reiki and SKHM, by Diane Ruth Shewmaker (WA: Celestial Wellspring Publications, 1999).

Anatomy of the Spirit: The Seven States of Power and Healing, by Caroline Myss, Ph.D. (NY: Harmony Press, 1996).

The Creative Journal: The Art of Finding Yourself, by Lucia Capacchione, Ph.D. (OH: Swallow Press/Ohio University Press, 1979).

Essential Reiki: A Complete Guide to an Ancient Healing Art, by Diane Stein (CA: The Crossing Press, Inc., 1996).

Flower Essence Repertory, by Patricia Kaminski and Richard Katz (CA: The Flower Essense Society, 1994 revised edition).

Hands of Light: A Guide to Healing Through the Human Energy Field, by Barbara Ann Brennan (NY: Bantam Books, 1987).

The Illustrated Encyclopedia of Natural Remedies, by C. Norman Shealy, M.D., Ph.D. (Dorset, England: Element Books Limited, 1998).

Iyashino Gendai Reiki-ho: Modern Reiki Method for Healing, by Hiroshi Doi (BC, Canada: Fraser Journal Publishing, 2000).

Love Is in the Earth: A Kaleidoscope of Crystals, by Melody (CO: Earth-Love Publishing House, 1995).

Magic and Medicine of Plants, by the editors of Reader's Digest (NY: Reader's Digest, 1986).

The Meditation Sourcebook: Meditation for Mortals, by Holly Sumner, Ph.D. (NY: McGraw-Hill, 1999).

The Power of Reiki: An Ancient Hands-on Healing Technique, by Tanmaya Honervogt (NY: Owl Books, 1998).

Quantum-Touch: The Power to Heal, by Richard Gordon (CA: North Atlantic Books, 2002).

Reiki and the Healing Buddha, by Maureen J. Kelly (WI: Lotus Press, 2001).

Reiki: A Way of Life, by Patrica Rose Upczak (CO: Synchronicity Publishing, 1999).

Reiki: Hawayo Takata's Story, by Helen J. Haberly (MD: Archedigm Publications, 1990).

Reiki: The Legacy of Dr. Usui, by Frank Arjava Petter (WI: Lotus Press, 1998).

Soul-Level Healing: Techniques to Peel Away the Layers, by Jillian Smith C.Ht.,C.M.H. (IA: Thinkers' Press, 1996).

The Spirit of Reiki: The Complete Handbook of the Reiki System, by Walter Lübeck, Frank Arjava Petter, and William Lee Rand (WI: Lotus Press, 2001).

Wheels of Light: Chakras, Auras, and the Healing Energy of the Body, by Rosalyn Bruyere (NY: Fireside, 1994).

Periodicals

Reiki Magazine International
✎ *www.reikimagazine.com/com*

Reiki News Magazine
✎ *www.spiritualone.com/WebStore/ReikiNews.html*

Online Connections

Reiki Associations

Australian Reiki Connection (ARC)
40 Jarvis Crescent
North Dandenong, Vic 3175, Australia
Phone: 03 9791 2564
help@australianreikiconnection.com.au
✍ *www.australianreikiconnection.com.au*

Canadian Reiki Association
P.O. Box 74072, Hillcrest RPO
Vancouver, BC, V5V 5C8, Canada
Phone: 867-835-7525
reiki@reiki.ca
✍ *www.reiki.ca*

The International Association of Reiki Professionals (IARP)
P.O. Box 104
Harrisville, NH 03450
Phone: 603-881-8838
info@iarp.org
✍ *www.iarp.org*

International Center for Reiki Training
21421 Hilltop St., #28
Southfield, MI 48034
Phone: 248-948-8112, 800-332-8112
center@reiki.org
✍ *www.reiki.org*

The John Harvey Gray Center for Reiki Healing
P.O. Box 696
Rindge, NH 03461-0696
Phone: 603-899-3288
lgray@reiki.mv.com
✍ *www.mv.com/ipusers/reiki/index.html*

The Radiance Technique International Association, Inc. (TRTIA)
P.O. Box 40570
St. Petersburg, FL 33743-0570
Phone: 813-347-2106, 888-878-7733
TRTIA@aol.com
✍ *www.trtia.org*

The Reiki Alliance
204 N. Chestnut Street
Kellogg, ID 83837
Phone: 208-783-3535
info@reikialliance.com
✍ *www.reikialliance.com*

The Reiki Association (TRA)
Cornbrook Bridge House, Clee Hill
Ludlow, Shropshire, SY8 3QQ, UK
Phone: +44 (0) 1270 812829
KateJones@reikiassociation.org.uk
✍ *www.reikiassociation.org.uk*

Reiki Center for Healing Arts
1764 Hamlet Street
San Mateo, CA 94403
Phone: 650-345-7666
revfranb@pacbell.net
✍ *http://reikifranbrown.com*

The Reiki Foundation
P.O. Box 362
Brewster, NY 10509-0362
Phone: 845-278-3038
asunam@msn.com
✍ *www.asunam.com/reiki_foundation.htm*

The Reiki Healing Connection
633 Isaac Frye Highway
Wilton, NH 03086
Phone: 603-654-2787, 888-REIKI-4-U
reiki@reikienergy.com
✍ *www.reikienergy.com*

Reiki Outreach International
P.O. Box 191156
San Diego, CA 92159-1156
ann@annieo.com
✍ *www.annieo.com/reikioutreach/id2.htm*

UK Reiki Federation
P.O. Box 1785
Andover, SP11 OWB, UK
Phone: +44 (0) 1264 773774
enquiry@reikifed.co.uk
✍ *www.reikifed.co.uk*

The United Kingdom Reiki Alliance
P.O. Box 114
Stowmarket, Suffolk, IP14 4WA, UK
Phone: +44 (0) 1449 673449
info@reikialliance.co.uk
✍ *www.reikialliance.co.uk*

Reiki Masters

Vincent Amador
✍ *www.reiki-do.org*

Fran Brown
Reiki Center for Healing Arts
1764 Hamlet Street
San Mateo, CA 94403
revfranb@pacbell.net
✍ *www.reikifranbrown.com*

Phyllis Lei Furumoto
✍ *www.usuireiki.com*

John Harvey Gray and Lourdes Gray
P.O. Box 696
Rindge, NH 03461-0696
lgray@reiki.mv.com
✍ *www.mv.com/ipusers/reiki*

Dave King
✍ *www.usui-do.org/~daveking/dave.html*

Light and Adonea
✍ *www.angelfire.com/az/SpiritMatters*

Walter Lübeck
✍ *www.rainbowreiki.net*

Mary Alexandra McFadyen
Reiki Outreach International
P.O. Box 191156
San Diego, CA 92159-1156
✍ *www.annieo.com/reikioutreach*

Paul Mitchell
✍ *www.usuireiki.com*

Frank Arjava Petter
✍ *www.reikidharma.com*

William Lee Rand
✍ *www.reiki.org/ReikiClasses/teachers/rand.html*

Barbara Weber Ray
The Radiance Technique International
    Association
P.O. Box 40570
St. Petersburg, FL 33743-0570
trtia@trtia.org
✍ *www.trtia.org*

Reverend Beverley Jean Voss
vosswood@team-national.com

Reiki Systems

Authentic Reiki
www.authenticreiki.org

Karuna Ki
Reiki Plain and Simple
http://angelreiki.nu

Karuna Reiki
The International Center for Reiki Training
www.reiki.org

Kundalini Reiki
Kundalini Mastery
www.kundalinireiki.com

Lightarian Reiki
Lightarian Institute
www.lightarian.com

Rainbow Reiki
Reiki-Do Institute
www.rainbowreiki.net

Raku Kai Reiki
http://angelreiki.nu

Reiki-Seichem and Gendai Reiki
www.reiki-seichem.com

Shamballa Reiki
Shamballa Healing
www.shamballahealing.com
www.members.aol.com/torcboy/shamballa.html

Tera-Mai Reiki Holistic Healing
http://teramaireiki.tripod.com
www.reikihealing.com.au

Transformational Reiki
Homepage of Steven and Karyn Mitchell
www.essex1.com/people/mitchell

Tummo Rei Ki
www.tummo.netfirms.com

Violet Flame Reiki
www.powerattunements.com

Wei Chi Tibetan Reiki
www.weboflight.com

Other Healing Modalities

Alexander Technique
www.alexandertechnique.com.au

Bowen Therapy
Gerri Shapiro
www.miraclepainrelief.com

Healing Touch
Healing Touch International, Inc.
www.healingtouch.net

Huna Healing
http://hunahealing.com

Johrei Healing
www.johreifoundation.org

Polarity Therapy
www.polaritytherapy.org

Pranic Healing
www.pranichealing.com

Quantum-Touch
✍ *www.quantumtouch.com*

Therapeutic Touch
✍ *www.therapeutic-touch.org*

Trager Approach
✍ *www.trager-us.org*

VortexHealing
✍ *www.vortexhealing.com*

Reiki Chats and Chatrooms

About.com Holistic Healing Chat
✍ *http://healing.about.com/mpchat.htm*

Access Reiki Chat
✍ *www.oznumberone.net/reiki-healing/reiki.chat.htm*

The Halls of Reiki Chat Room
✍ *http://pub18.bravenet.com/chat/show.php/154 4305713*

ICQ List—Healing Across the Internet
✍ *www.create.org/list.htm*

Light and Adonea's Reiki Chat
✍ *www.geocities.com/HotSprings/9434/lachat.html*

Reiki Cafe
✍ *www.nexuscafe.com/bin/home.cgi/Home/reiki*

Reiki Fitness Chatroom
✍ *www.reikifitness.com/QuickChat.htm*

Reiki Massage Conference Room
✍ *www.alt-med-ed.com/practices/reiki.htm*

Subtle Energies Reiki Chat
✍ *www.reikiconnect.com/reikichat.htm*

Violet Energy of Reiki Chat
✍ *http://reiki.msk.ru/english/chat.html*

Reiki Message Boards

About.com Reiki Forums
✍ *http://forums.about.com/ab-healing2/start/*

Reiki 4 All Forums
✍ *www.reikicentrum.nl/reiki4all/forums/*

Reiki Cafe Message Board
✍ *www.nexuscafe.com/bin/bbs.cgi/ShowBoardList/reiki*

ReikiOne Message Center
✍ *www.reikione.com/cgi-bin/forum.cgi*

Reiki UseNet and News Groups

Avalon's Vibrational Healing Mailing List
✍ *www.home.aone.net.au/crystalhealing*

Yahoo Reiki Groups
✍ *http://dir.groups.yahoo.com/dir/1600060843*

Usenet News Groups, Reiki
✍ *news:alt.healing.reiki*
✍ *news:own.health.reiki*
✍ *news:sff.people.reikihaven*

Reiki Web Rings

Angel Reiki
✍ *http://T.webring.com/hub?ring=angelreiki*

Ascension Reiki
✍ *http://L.webring.com/hub?ring=ascensionreikiwe*

Grassroots Reiki
✍ *http://L.webring.com/hub?ring=grassrootsreiki*

Mayan Reiki

✍ *http://K.webring.com/hub?ring=mayanreiki*

Reiki 4 All Web Ring

✍ *www.xs4all.nl/~remy/webring.html*

The Reiki Master WebRing

✍ *http://Q.webring.com/hub?ring=Buddha*

The Reiki Teacher Network

✍ *http://P.webring.com/hub?ring=thereikiteachern*

ReikiOne.com WebRing

✍ *www.reikione.com*

World Wide Reiki Ring

✍ *http://E.webring.com/hub?ring=reikiring*

Reiki Practitioner Directories

About.com Holistic Healing

Reiki Practitioner Locator; International Reiki Directory

✍*http://healing.about.com/library/blreiki_internl.htm*

Centre of Peaceful Light Reiki

Reiki Masters and Practitioners

✍ *www.reiki.com/rmpracts.html*

Find-It-Hypermart

International Directory of Reiki Practitioners/Therapists

✍ *http://find-it.hypermart.net/reiki.htm*

IARP

International Association of Reiki Professionals

✍ *http://data.iarp.org/members*

Mind Body Spirit Directory

✍ *http://w3.one.net/~source*

ReikiOne.com

ReikiOne Practitioner/Teacher Directory

✍ *www.reikione.com/cgi-bin/directory.cgi*

Other Related Web Resources

Alexandria Reiki Centre

✍ *www.alexandriahealing.co.uk*

Healing Rays

www.healing-rays.com

Highly Sensitive People

✍ *http://highlysensitivepeople.com*

Japanese Kanji

✍ *www.thejapanesepage.com*

Law of Life Books

Ascended Master Kuthumi

✍ *www.lawoflife.com*

Sacred Spaces

✍ *www.sacredspaceswa.com*

Reiki in Hospitals

✍ *www.srpt.org*

The Reiki Ryoho Gakkai

✍ *www.usuireiki.fsnet.co.uk*

The Reiki Threshold

✍ *www.threshold.ca*

Solar Raven

✍ *www.solarraven.com*

Index

THE EVERYTHING SERIES!

BUSINESS & PERSONAL FINANCE

Everything® Accounting Book
Everything® Budgeting Book
Everything® Business Planning Book
Everything® Coaching and Mentoring Book
Everything® Fundraising Book
Everything® Get Out of Debt Book
Everything® Grant Writing Book
Everything® Guide to Personal Finance for Single Mothers
Everything® Home-Based Business Book, 2nd Ed.
Everything® Homebuying Book, 2nd Ed.
Everything® Homeselling Book, 2nd Ed.
Everything® Improve Your Credit Book
Everything® Investing Book, 2nd Ed.
Everything® Landlording Book
Everything® Leadership Book
Everything® Managing People Book, 2nd Ed.
Everything® Negotiating Book
Everything® Online Auctions Book
Everything® Online Business Book
Everything® Personal Finance Book
Everything® Personal Finance in Your 20s and 30s Book
Everything® Project Management Book
Everything® Real Estate Investing Book
Everything® Retirement Planning Book
Everything® Robert's Rules Book, $7.95
Everything® Selling Book
Everything® Start Your Own Business Book, 2nd Ed.
Everything® Wills & Estate Planning Book

COOKING

Everything® Barbecue Cookbook
Everything® Bartender's Book, $9.95
Everything® Cheese Book
Everything® Chinese Cookbook
Everything® Classic Recipes Book
Everything® Cocktail Parties and Drinks Book
Everything® College Cookbook
Everything® Cooking for Baby and Toddler Book
Everything® Cooking for Two Cookbook
Everything® Diabetes Cookbook
Everything® Easy Gourmet Cookbook
Everything® Fondue Cookbook
Everything® Fondue Party Book
Everything® Gluten-Free Cookbook
Everything® Glycemic Index Cookbook
Everything® Grilling Cookbook

Everything® Healthy Meals in Minutes Cookbook
Everything® Holiday Cookbook
Everything® Indian Cookbook
Everything® Italian Cookbook
Everything® Low-Carb Cookbook
Everything® Low-Fat High-Flavor Cookbook
Everything® Low-Salt Cookbook
Everything® Meals for a Month Cookbook
Everything® Mediterranean Cookbook
Everything® Mexican Cookbook
Everything® No Trans Fat Cookbook
Everything® One-Pot Cookbook
Everything® Pizza Cookbook
Everything® Quick and Easy 30-Minute, 5-Ingredient Cookbook
Everything® Quick Meals Cookbook
Everything® Slow Cooker Cookbook
Everything® Slow Cooking for a Crowd Cookbook
Everything® Soup Cookbook
Everything® Stir-Fry Cookbook
Everything® Tex-Mex Cookbook
Everything® Thai Cookbook
Everything® Vegetarian Cookbook
Everything® Wild Game Cookbook
Everything® Wine Book, 2nd Ed.

GAMES

Everything® 15-Minute Sudoku Book, $9.95
Everything® 30-Minute Sudoku Book, $9.95
Everything® Blackjack Strategy Book
Everything® Brain Strain Book, $9.95
Everything® Bridge Book
Everything® Card Games Book
Everything® Card Tricks Book, $9.95
Everything® Casino Gambling Book, 2nd Ed.
Everything® Chess Basics Book
Everything® Craps Strategy Book
Everything® Crossword and Puzzle Book
Everything® Crossword Challenge Book
Everything® Crosswords for the Beach Book, $9.95
Everything® Cryptograms Book, $9.95
Everything® Easy Crosswords Book
Everything® Easy Kakuro Book, $9.95
Everything® Easy Large Print Crosswords Book
Everything® Games Book, 2nd Ed.
Everything® Giant Sudoku Book, $9.95
Everything® Kakuro Challenge Book, $9.95
Everything® Large-Print Crossword Challenge Book

Everything® Large-Print Crosswords Book
Everything® Lateral Thinking Puzzles Book, $9.95
Everything® Mazes Book
Everything® Movie Crosswords Book, $9.95
Everything® Online Poker Book, $12.95
Everything® Pencil Puzzles Book, $9.95
Everything® Poker Strategy Book
Everything® Pool & Billiards Book
Everything® Sports Crosswords Book, $9.95
Everything® Test Your IQ Book, $9.95
Everything® Texas Hold 'Em Book, $9.95
Everything® Travel Crosswords Book, $9.95
Everything® Word Games Challenge Book
Everything® Word Scramble Book
Everything® Word Search Book

HEALTH

Everything® Alzheimer's Book
Everything® Diabetes Book
Everything® Health Guide to Adult Bipolar Disorder
Everything® Health Guide to Controlling Anxiety
Everything® Health Guide to Fibromyalgia
Everything® Health Guide to Postpartum Care
Everything® Health Guide to Thyroid Disease
Everything® Hypnosis Book
Everything® Low Cholesterol Book
Everything® Massage Book
Everything® Menopause Book
Everything® Nutrition Book
Everything® Reflexology Book
Everything® Stress Management Book

HISTORY

Everything® American Government Book
Everything® American History Book, 2nd Ed.
Everything® Civil War Book
Everything® Freemasons Book
Everything® Irish History & Heritage Book
Everything® Middle East Book

HOBBIES

Everything® Candlemaking Book
Everything® Cartooning Book
Everything® Coin Collecting Book
Everything® Drawing Book
Everything® Family Tree Book, 2nd Ed.
Everything® Knitting Book
Everything® Knots Book
Everything® Photography Book

Everything® Quilting Book
Everything® Scrapbooking Book
Everything® Sewing Book
Everything® Soapmaking Book, 2nd Ed.
Everything® Woodworking Book

HOME IMPROVEMENT

Everything® Feng Shui Book
Everything® Feng Shui Decluttering Book, $9.95
Everything® Fix-It Book
Everything® Home Decorating Book
Everything® Home Storage Solutions Book
Everything® Homebuilding Book
Everything® Organize Your Home Book

KIDS' BOOKS

All titles are $7.95

Everything® Kids' Animal Puzzle & Activity Book
Everything® Kids' Baseball Book, 4th Ed.
Everything® Kids' Bible Trivia Book
Everything® Kids' Bugs Book
Everything® Kids' Cars and Trucks Puzzle
 & Activity Book
Everything® Kids' Christmas Puzzle
 & Activity Book
Everything® Kids' Cookbook
Everything® Kids' Crazy Puzzles Book
Everything® Kids' Dinosaurs Book
Everything® Kids' First Spanish Puzzle and
 Activity Book
Everything® Kids' Gross Cookbook
Everything® Kids' Gross Hidden Pictures Book
Everything® Kids' Gross Jokes Book
Everything® Kids' Gross Mazes Book
Everything® Kids' Gross Puzzle and
 Activity Book
Everything® Kids' Halloween Puzzle
 & Activity Book
Everything® Kids' Hidden Pictures Book
Everything® Kids' Horses Book
Everything® Kids' Joke Book
Everything® Kids' Knock Knock Book
Everything® Kids' Learning Spanish Book
Everything® Kids' Math Puzzles Book
Everything® Kids' Mazes Book
Everything® Kids' Money Book
Everything® Kids' Nature Book
Everything® Kids' Pirates Puzzle and Activity Book
Everything® Kids' Presidents Book
Everything® Kids' Princess Puzzle and Activity Book
Everything® Kids' Puzzle Book
Everything® Kids' Riddles & Brain Teasers Book
Everything® Kids' Science Experiments Book
Everything® Kids' Sharks Book
Everything® Kids' Soccer Book
Everything® Kids' States Book
Everything® Kids' Travel Activity Book

KIDS' STORY BOOKS

Everything® Fairy Tales Book

LANGUAGE

Everything® Conversational Japanese Book with
 CD, $19.95
Everything® French Grammar Book
Everything® French Phrase Book, $9.95
Everything® French Verb Book, $9.95
Everything® German Practice Book with CD,
 $19.95
Everything® Inglés Book
**Everything® Intermediate Spanish Book with
 CD, $19.95**
**Everything® Learning Brazilian Portuguese
 Book with CD, $19.95**
Everything® Learning French Book
Everything® Learning German Book
Everything® Learning Italian Book
Everything® Learning Latin Book
**Everything® Learning Spanish Book with
 CD, 2nd Edition, $19.95**
Everything® Russian Practice Book with CD, $19.95
Everything® Sign Language Book
Everything® Spanish Grammar Book
Everything® Spanish Phrase Book, $9.95
Everything® Spanish Practice Book
 with CD, $19.95
Everything® Spanish Verb Book, $9.95
Everything® Speaking Mandarin Chinese Book
 with CD, $19.95

MUSIC

Everything® Drums Book with CD, $19.95
**Everything® Guitar Book with CD, 2nd
 Edition, $19.95**
Everything® Guitar Chords Book with CD, $19.95
Everything® Home Recording Book
Everything® Music Theory Book with CD, $19.95
Everything® Reading Music Book with CD, $19.95
Everything® Rock & Blues Guitar Book
 with CD, $19.95
**Everything® Rock and Blues Piano Book
 with CD, $19.95**
Everything® Songwriting Book

NEW AGE

Everything® Astrology Book, 2nd Ed.
Everything® Birthday Personology Book
Everything® Dreams Book, 2nd Ed.
Everything® Love Signs Book, $9.95
Everything® Numerology Book
Everything® Paganism Book
Everything® Palmistry Book
Everything® Psychic Book
Everything® Reiki Book

Everything® Sex Signs Book, $9.95
Everything® Tarot Book, 2nd Ed.
Everything® Toltec Wisdom Book
Everything® Wicca and Witchcraft Book

PARENTING

Everything® Baby Names Book, 2nd Ed.
Everything® Baby Shower Book
Everything® Baby's First Year Book
Everything® Birthing Book
Everything® Breastfeeding Book
Everything® Father-to-Be Book
Everything® Father's First Year Book
Everything® Get Ready for Baby Book
Everything® Get Your Baby to Sleep Book, $9.95
Everything® Getting Pregnant Book
Everything® Guide to Raising a One-Year-Old
Everything® Guide to Raising a Two-Year-Old
Everything® Homeschooling Book
Everything® Mother's First Year Book
**Everything® Parent's Guide to Childhood
 Illnesses**
Everything® Parent's Guide to Children
 and Divorce
Everything® Parent's Guide to Children
 with ADD/ADHD
Everything® Parent's Guide to Children
 with Asperger's Syndrome
Everything® Parent's Guide to Children
 with Autism
Everything® Parent's Guide to Children with
 Bipolar Disorder
**Everything® Parent's Guide to Children with
 Depression**
Everything® Parent's Guide to Children
 with Dyslexia
**Everything® Parent's Guide to Children with
 Juvenile Diabetes**
Everything® Parent's Guide to Positive Discipline
Everything® Parent's Guide to Raising a
 Successful Child
Everything® Parent's Guide to Raising Boys
Everything® Parent's Guide to Raising Girls
Everything® Parent's Guide to Raising Siblings
Everything® Parent's Guide to Sensory
 Integration Disorder
Everything® Parent's Guide to Tantrums
Everything® Parent's Guide to the Strong-Willed
 Child
Everything® Parenting a Teenager Book
Everything® Potty Training Book, $9.95
Everything® Pregnancy Book, 3rd Ed.
Everything® Pregnancy Fitness Book
Everything® Pregnancy Nutrition Book
Everything® Pregnancy Organizer, 2nd Ed., $16.95
Everything® Toddler Activities Book
Everything® Toddler Book

Everything® Tween Book
Everything® Twins, Triplets, and More Book

PETS

Everything® Aquarium Book
Everything® Boxer Book
Everything® Cat Book, 2nd Ed.
Everything® Chihuahua Book
Everything® Dachshund Book
Everything® Dog Book
Everything® Dog Health Book
Everything® Dog Obedience Book
Everything® Dog Owner's Organizer, $16.95
Everything® Dog Training and Tricks Book
Everything® German Shepherd Book
Everything® Golden Retriever Book
Everything® Horse Book
Everything® Horse Care Book
Everything® Horseback Riding Book
Everything® Labrador Retriever Book
Everything® Poodle Book
Everything® Pug Book
Everything® Puppy Book
Everything® Rottweiler Book
Everything® Small Dogs Book
Everything® Tropical Fish Book
Everything® Yorkshire Terrier Book

REFERENCE

Everything® American Presidents Book
Everything® Blogging Book
Everything® Build Your Vocabulary Book
Everything® Car Care Book
Everything® Classical Mythology Book
Everything® Da Vinci Book
Everything® Divorce Book
Everything® Einstein Book
Everything® Enneagram Book
Everything® Etiquette Book, 2nd Ed.
Everything® Inventions and Patents Book
Everything® Mafia Book
Everything® Philosophy Book
Everything® Pirates Book
Everything® Psychology Book

RELIGION

Everything® Angels Book
Everything® Bible Book
Everything® Buddhism Book
Everything® Catholicism Book
Everything® Christianity Book
Everything® Gnostic Gospels Book
Everything® History of the Bible Book
Everything® Jesus Book

Everything® Jewish History & Heritage Book
Everything® Judaism Book
Everything® Kabbalah Book
Everything® Koran Book
Everything® Mary Book
Everything® Mary Magdalene Book
Everything® Prayer Book
Everything® Saints Book, 2nd Ed.
Everything® Torah Book
Everything® Understanding Islam Book
Everything® World's Religions Book
Everything® Zen Book

SCHOOL & CAREERS

Everything® Alternative Careers Book
Everything® Career Tests Book
Everything® College Major Test Book
Everything® College Survival Book, 2nd Ed.
Everything® Cover Letter Book, 2nd Ed.
Everything® Filmmaking Book
Everything® Get-a-Job Book, 2nd Ed.
Everything® Guide to Being a Paralegal
Everything® Guide to Being a Personal Trainer
Everything® Guide to Being a Real Estate Agent
Everything® Guide to Being a Sales Rep
Everything® Guide to Careers in Health Care
Everything® Guide to Careers in Law Enforcement
Everything® Guide to Government Jobs
Everything® Guide to Starting and Running a Restaurant
Everything® Job Interview Book
Everything® New Nurse Book
Everything® New Teacher Book
Everything® Paying for College Book
Everything® Practice Interview Book
Everything® Resume Book, 2nd Ed.
Everything® Study Book

SELF-HELP

Everything® Dating Book, 2nd Ed.
Everything® Great Sex Book
Everything® Self-Esteem Book
Everything® Tantric Sex Book

SPORTS & FITNESS

Everything® Easy Fitness Book
Everything® Running Book
Everything® Weight Training Book

TRAVEL

Everything® Family Guide to Cruise Vacations
Everything® Family Guide to Hawaii
Everything® Family Guide to Las Vegas, 2nd Ed.
Everything® Family Guide to Mexico
Everything® Family Guide to New York City, 2nd Ed.
Everything® Family Guide to RV Travel & Campgrounds
Everything® Family Guide to the Caribbean
Everything® Family Guide to the Walt Disney World Resort®, Universal Studios®, and Greater Orlando, 4th Ed.
Everything® Family Guide to Timeshares
Everything® Family Guide to Washington D.C., 2nd Ed.

WEDDINGS

Everything® Bachelorette Party Book, $9.95
Everything® Bridesmaid Book, $9.95
Everything® Destination Wedding Book
Everything® Elopement Book, $9.95
Everything® Father of the Bride Book, $9.95
Everything® Groom Book, $9.95
Everything® Mother of the Bride Book, $9.95
Everything® Outdoor Wedding Book
Everything® Wedding Book, 3rd Ed.
Everything® Wedding Checklist, $9.95
Everything® Wedding Etiquette Book, $9.95
Everything® Wedding Organizer, 2nd Ed., $16.95
Everything® Wedding Shower Book, $9.95
Everything® Wedding Vows Book, $9.95
Everything® Wedding Workout Book
Everything® Weddings on a Budget Book, $9.95

WRITING

Everything® Creative Writing Book
Everything® Get Published Book, 2nd Ed.
Everything® Grammar and Style Book
Everything® Guide to Magazine Writing
Everything® Guide to Writing a Book Proposal
Everything® Guide to Writing a Novel
Everything® Guide to Writing Children's Books
Everything® Guide to Writing Copy
Everything® Guide to Writing Research Papers
Everything® Screenwriting Book
Everything® Writing Poetry Book
Everything® Writing Well Book